£15-00

Political anatomy of the body

Medical knowledge in Britain in the twentieth century

Political anatomy of the body

Medical knowledge in Britain in the twentieth century

DAVID ARMSTRONG
Guy's Hospital Medical School

CAMBRIDGE UNIVERSITY PRESS
Cambridge
London New York New Rochelle
Melbourne Sydney

Published by the Press Syndicate of the University of Cambridge
The Pitt Building, Trumpington Street, Cambridge CB2 1RP
32 East 57th Street, New York, NY 10022, USA
296 Beaconsfield Parade, Middle Park, Melbourne 3206, Australia

First published 1983

Printed in Great Britain at
the University Press, Cambridge

Library of Congress catalogue card number: 82-9546

British Library cataloguing in publication data

Armstrong, David
Political anatomy of the body.
1. Social medicine – Great Britain
I. Title
362.1'0941 RA418

ISBN 0 521 24746 2

CE

for Pauline

Contents

Acknowledgements

I am grateful for the guidance and encouragement of Margot Jefferys who acted as my supervisor for the thesis on which this book is based. I am also indebted to those many colleagues within medical sociology who have made helpful comments on the various papers and drafts which have gone to make up the final work. Perhaps I should mention in particular the valuable critical points made by Bill Arney, Robert Dingwall, Gordon Horobin and Peter Miller.

My thanks are also due to Carol Butterfield who did all the typing with her usual skill and forebearance, and to Cambridge University Press, particularly Sheila Shepherd for valuable editorial help.

Preface

I doubt if it ever occurred to me or my fellow medical students that the human body which we dissected and examined was other than a stable experience. It was therefore with considerable surprise that years later I learned that it was only since the end of the eighteenth century that disease had been localised to specific organs and tissues, and that bodies had been subjected to the rigours of clinical examination.

At first it seemed strange to me how the apparent obviousness of disease and its manifestations inside the body had eluded scientific discovery for so long. How had pre-Enlightenment generations failed to see the clearly differentiated organs and tissues of the body? Or failed to link patient symptoms with the existence of localised pathological processes? Or failed to apply the most rudimentary diagnostic techniques of physical examination? My disbelief grew until it occurred to me that perhaps I was asking the wrong questions: the problem was not how something which is so obvious today had remained hidden for so long, but how the body had become so evident in the first place. In dissecting and examining bodies I had come to take for granted that what I saw was obvious. I had thought that medical knowledge simply described the body. I argue in this book that the relationship is more complex, that medical knowledge both describes and constructs the body as an invariate biological reality.

It was the work of Michel Foucault which offered me a means of grasping the relationship between medical knowledge and its object, the body. For Foucault, the concept of the body which emerged at the end of the eighteenth century – discrete, objective, passive, analysable – was the effect as well as the object of medical inquiry. The first chapter of this book attempts to set out more fully Foucault's arguments, particularly as they pertain to events during the late eighteenth century: I hope that I have neither over-simplified nor misreported. I should, however, point out that Foucault's evidence is drawn primarily from French sources and many of the changes he documents – such as the emergence of individualism – may have occurred over a longer time period in the Anglo-Saxon world. Nevertheless, I remain impressed with the general thrust of his argument and the details of his method, and there seems little doubt, at least so far as medicine is concerned, that Parisian hospitals at the end of the eighteenth century formed the epicentre of a medical revolution.

Following this introductory chapter the book deals almost exclusively with medical writings in Britain in the twentieth century and pursues an argument that this period has witnessed a further fundamental reformulation of the nature and identity of the human body. Chapters 2, 3 and 4 deal with events prior to World War II: chapter 2 develops the general model I employ, while chapters 3 and 4 offer, in the development of the neuroses and of social medicine, particular illustrations. Chapter 5 outlines the development of the survey as a medical technique during the war years, and the following five chapters cover the post-war emergence of the disciplines of paediatrics, psychiatry, general practice, geriatrics and community medicine. The penultimate chapter, through a documentation of the doctor–patient relationship during the period, attempts to show how these various medical events have served to fabricate, not, as in the nineteenth century, a discrete, passive, physical body, but an essentially relative and subjective one.

I might add that while the book deals with medical knowledge in the twentieth century it is not meant to be a history of events. I am trying to deal with what Foucault terms 'conditions of possibility'. I am therefore not concerned with whether the medical perceptions which I document were in any sense correct or typical but rather at what point a thought became thinkable. I hope therefore that the argument of the book is applicable outside the narrow geographical confines of Britain. To this end, in the final chapter – which acts as a postscript to the general thesis – I have tried to show the parallel points in the human sciences, as they developed in the Anglo-Saxon world during the twentieth century, when particular techniques, approaches and knowledges of the body became possible.

1

The clinical gaze

> For us the human body defines, by natural right, the space of origin and of distribution of disease: a space whose lines, volumes, surfaces, and routes are laid down, in accordance with a now familiar geometry, by the anatomical atlas. But this order of the solid, visible body is only one way – in all likelihood neither the first, nor the most fundamental – in which one spatializes disease. There have been, and will be, other distributions of illness.
>
> Michel Foucault: *The birth of the clinic*[1]

The anatomical atlas stands between ignorance and medical knowledge. By means of the atlas a confusing mass of cells, tissues and organs is given a pattern: specific structures are indicated by means of arrows and labels, the relationships between organs and tissues are made clear by the use of different colours and the great systems of the body are identified by overlying transparencies. With the aid of these various techniques of illustration the atlas depicts the organisation and solidity of the three-dimensional body on the two-dimensional page; it enables the interior of the body to be differentiated and deciphered to the point at which an observer is able – from the outside without dissection – to read the internal structures and their changes. The atlas renders the body transparent; it is a means of making the body *legible* to an observing eye.

There was a time of course, before the atlas, when the body could not be read with such clarity. It was not that the body was illegible, more that there were different languages by which it was read – those of the soldier, the astrologer, the lay healer (many undoubtedly never committed to paper). Foucault, for example, describes an eighteenth-century French physician who treated a hysteric by making her take frequent baths and then reported seeing 'membranous tissues like pieces of damp parchment ... peel away with some slight discomfort, and these were passed daily with the urine', or the intestines 'peeled off their internal tunics, which we saw emerge from the rectum'.[2] In terms of the twentieth-century anatomical atlas which informs the gaze deep into the body such observations are virtually unintelligible because, at the moment the modern atlas made its appearance, the old languages, the ancient ways of seeing, disappeared. In their place came a more penetrating gaze that used the new techniques of observations, palpation, percussion and auscultation and made the deepest recesses of the body transparent to the medical eye.

The fact that the body became legible does not imply that some invariate biological reality was finally revealed to medical enquiry. The body was only legible in that there existed in the new clinical techniques a language by which it could be read. The anatomical atlas directs attention to certain structures, certain similarities, certain systems, and not others and in so doing forms a set of rules for reading the body and for making it intelligible. In this sense the reality of the body is only established by the observing eye that reads it. The atlas enables the anatomy student, when faced with the undifferentiated amorphous mass of the body, to see certain things and ignore others. In effect, what the student sees is not the atlas as a representation of the body but the body as a representation of the atlas.

The atlas is therefore a means of interpreting the body, of seeing its form and nature and establishing its reality. The modern body of the patient, which has become the unquestioned object of clinical practice, has no social existence prior to those same clinical techniques being exercised upon it. It is as if the medical gaze, in which is encompassed all the techniques, languages and assumptions of modern medicine, establishes by its authority and penetration an observable and analysable space in which is crystallised that apparently solid figure – which has now become so familiar – the discrete human body.

The analysis of the way the body is seen, described and constructed, Foucault suggests, might be called 'political anatomy'.[3] It is political because the changes in the way the body is described are not the consequences of some random effects or progressive enlightenment but are based on certain mechanisms of power which, since the eighteenth century, have pervaded the body and continue to hold it in their grasp. From that time the body has been the point on which and from which power has been exercised.

Mechanisms of power

Towards the end of the eighteenth century medical men started to subject their patients to physical examination. The basis of this change in medical procedure was the newly discovered pathological anatomy by which diseases became localisable in the body of the patient: in place of the constantly shifting symptoms in the patient's history medicine pin-pointed pathology in the interior of the body and used the ever more detailed methods of the examination to diagnose it. Contemporaneously a change occurred in the regime of criminal punishment: from being subjected to torture, pillorying and public display the criminal became incarcerated and subjected to continuous surveillance behind the high walls of the prison.

Foucault argues that these changes in the way the body was treated were not coincidental but reflected a new political anatomy: 'the classical age discovered the body as object and target of power'.[4] Throughout European society during this period the body became treated 'as something docile that could be subjected, used, transformed and improved'. The body became surrounded and invested with various techniques of detail which analysed, monitored and fabricated it. Architectural space became governed by the need to assign particular places to particular individuals (and, conversely, individuals to particular places). The individual was no longer placed in a fixed social place but in a rank which stressed relations of positions. Bodily activities were temporally ordered. The timetable, for a long time used in monastic communities to preclude idleness, was more widely introduced to establish rhythms, impose particular occupations and regulate the cycles of repetition in schools, workshops, prisons and hospitals. These different ways of seeing bodies served to establish a true political economy of the corporal in which time, detail and gesture were broken down into their component parts, analysed and reconstituted to exact from coordinated and disciplined bodies more than the sum of their separate contributions.

These various techniques of analysis that invested the body all involved surveillance: bodies had to be inspected to judge their status, they had to be analysed to identify their deficits and they had to be monitored to evaluate their functioning. The importance of surveillance is illustrated in particular in the various techniques of examination that emerged to prominence in the eighteenth century such as the clinical examination in the hospital, the inspection in the prison, the test in the school and the military inspection in the barracks. Together, these procedures served to ensure that the person under observation was the object of a detailed analysis.

Foucault suggests that these various techniques represented different aspects of a disciplinary apparatus. Discipline involves attention to fine detail, to strict monitoring and to the object of the disciplinary regime – the individual body – being trained to function with coordination and efficiency: through discipline, surveillance fabricates a manipulable body. Discipline is a mechanism that invests the body of whoever is observed, transforming an unorganised and incoherent being into an efficient structure. The army, for example, took untrained bodies and, through analysis of bodily movements in the routines of drill or the regular surveillance of parade-ground inspections and hierarchies of observation, succeeded in creating a disciplined soldier. The disciplinary apparatus was a creative technology which served to fabricate discrete individuals. The late eighteenth century saw the separate analysis and documentation of the body, from the case history in medicine to the appearance of ordinary people, in that new literary form, the novel; it was also marked by the first appearance of the word and notion of 'individualism'.

The observer, who through surveillance functioned to fabricate these individual identities, was neither unique nor important. Discipline depended not so much on a person as on an observing gaze. It mattered little who the observer was, more that he functioned as a component in a unified observation. 'The perfect disciplinary apparatus', Foucault notes, 'would make it possible for a single gaze to see everything constantly.' The configuration of power in a disciplinary regime was simply the relationship between an individualised body and a disembodied gaze. Power, in this sense, is not a thing, it is not something that is 'acquired, seized or shared, something that one holds on to or allows to slip away'.[5] Power is simply a shorthand for describing a certain 'strategic relation' in a given society. Thus power in the hierarchised surveillance of the disciplinary techniques 'functions as a piece of machinery. And, although it [has] a head, it is the apparatus as a whole that produces "power" and distributes individuals in the permanent and continuous field.'

Under the old regime the mechanism of power was represented by sovereignty in which the population was subjected to the 'spectacle of power'. Sovereignty functioned through being visible to those on whom it had its effects: the royal presence was signified by outward shows of ostentation, the ceremony and the ritual, palaces, processions, public displays and marks of allegiance. In contrast, disciplinary power inverted the principle of visibility; it required, not the visibility of itself, but of its target – and that target was the individual body which became at the same time both object and effect of the disciplinary gaze. There had of course been 'individuals' in previous societies but, in that they emerged under a regime of sovereign power, they had been marked out by privilege, ritual, heroics and ceremonies. In the disciplinary regime, on the other hand, individualisation commenced at the 'bottom' bringing 'ordinary individuality – the everyday individuality of everybody – [from] below the threshold of description'.

With the new 'micro-physics' of power, in which the individual body became the target and effect of a ubiquitous and calculating gaze, the field of knowledge and human understanding was reformulated. It became possible to imagine a docile workforce, a disciplined army, a growing child and a medicine that analysed and investigated bodies. The ordinary individual emerged in, and was fabricated by, the discourse of the age; and the study of the individual in the form of the human sciences became a possibility.

Panopticism

Foucault suggests that the particular configuration of an individuated, analysed body and a disembodied gaze found its near-perfect representation in Bentham's plans for an ideal prison, the Panopticon. The design of the Panopticon was of a building arranged as a ring, at the centre of which was a tower. The peripheral building was divided into cells; each cell had two windows, an outer one to allow light to fall on the inmate and an inner one to allow a guard in the central tower to observe the inmate's actions. The central tower was pierced by large windows opening onto the inner side of the peripheral ring. These windows allowed the guard full visibility of the prisoners but because they were also shuttered they prevented the prisoner being aware of when and by whom he was being observed. Each cell was thus 'like so many cages, so many small theatres, in which each actor is alone, perfectly individualised and constantly visible'.

As disciplinary power spread throughout European society at the end of the eighteenth century the Panopticon served as an architectural model for all those agencies which sought to analyse and improve the efficiency of individual bodies. New institutions emerged with high external walls – schools, hospitals, barracks, prisons and workshops – but whose internal arrangements permitted constant visibility of their inmates to an ever-probing gaze. 'The crowd, a compact mass, a locus of multiple exchanges, individualities merging together, a collective effect is abolished and replaced by a collection of separate individualities.'

The panoptic vision was not simply a technique by which those in authority could repress a population; nor can it be analysed in terms of the 'social control' of those deviants and outcasts of capitalist society who threatened to undermine the social order. The Panopticon was not a dream building in which men and women were enslaved but 'the diagram of a mechanism of power reduced to its ideal form'. To see the Panopticon as an institution of repression is to treat power as something that forbids and alienates. The Panopticon represented a creative arrangement of power which fabricated an individual body – that very body which was to be the point on which repression could be exercised and into which ideologies could be inscribed, but, nonetheless, a body which had no existence prior to its crystallisation in the space delineated by a monitoring gaze.

In part, because panoptic surveillance works through a system of 'inverted visibility', the nature of power, of its basis in an ideal optical arrangement, has tended to remain hidden and even concealed. Thus the anatomical atlas, for all its short history, would claim that the body which it describes is a universal and fixed biological entity. Even those disciplines which would disclaim a biological basis still accept the *a priori* existence of an individualised analysable body. Yet, within the discourse of all these various disciplines of the individual, there lies an imprint of a body which was at the same time both the object of analysis and its effect.

It is apparent, as Foucault observes, that late in the eighteenth century medicine began to see a body which had a new anatomy. This body appears to have been discrete because it was recorded in separate case notes; it was accessible because at this time medicine began to use methods of physical examination; it was analysable because pathology became localisable to a distinct point within the body; it was passive because the patient's personal history was relegated from its primary position as the key to the diagnosis to a preliminary; and it was subjected to evaluation because patients were moved from the natural locus of the home to the neutral domain of the hospital. Thus, every time medicine had cause to deploy its new techniques and treat an illness, it drew an outline of a particular anatomy, a docile body. At first the procedure was unsure and the outline hazy but with time and with refinement the shape became more clear. As the nineteenth century progressed each and every consultation of the new pathological medicine functioned to imprint, by its sheer repetition, the reality of a specific anatomy on a social conscience.

In a sense the true inheritance of this period is the anatomical atlas which proclaims on every page the solid, invariate reality of the body. Armed with this truth it becomes possible to view the events of the late eighteenth century as enlightenment: the abandonment of old superstitions, the laying to rest of moral qualms about the post-mortem and physical examination of the body, the brilliance of scientific advance, the technological breakthrough of the hospital. But there remains another anatomy whose truth is not to be discovered in the bright illumination of the dissecting room but in the dusty texts of forgotten knowledge. Therein lies the outline of a body that was not fashioned long ago in an East African rift valley but relatively recently in a medical gaze; a body that became intimately legible at the end of the eighteenth century, a body whose reality and transparency was consolidated in the nineteenth century, a body whose existence gave rise to and was sustained by myriad techniques ranging from the laws of cellular function to the great strategies of liberalism and individual contract.

In the twentieth century the diagram of power is rearranged. The medical gaze, which had for over a century analysed the microscopic detail of the individual body, began to move to the undifferentiated space between bodies and there proceeded to forge a new political anatomy.

2

The new hygiene of the Dispensary

In 1887, following the failure of the citizenry of Edinburgh to found a special hospital for tuberculosis, Dr Robert Philip opened a tuberculosis dispensary in Bank Street. In part, this dispensary functioned as an out-patient clinic to which patients with tuberculosis were referred for treatment; but it also arranged for a staff of nurses to visit the homes of patients so as to discover their needs, to report on their circumstances, to act as a conduit for charitable agencies, to report on contacts and to teach the healthy way of life. With all this activity the dispensary 'came to resemble the committee rooms of a general election where information is collected and distributed, work arranged and timorous supporters stimulated to duty'.[1]

The Edinburgh dispensary prospered and the idea spread. A Central Fund for the Promotion of the Dispensaries System was formed and started operating tuberculosis dispensaries in London in 1911. The Departmental Committee on Tuberculosis, established in the wake of the 1911 National Health Insurance Act, officially endorsed the concept and suggested that metropolitan borough councils should run and coordinate the growing number of privately sponsored dispensaries.[2] The Departmental Committee argued that the dispensary should be a model for the care and treatment of tuberculosis patients in as much as it offered a complete service. The dispensary was a receiving house and centre of diagnosis; besides confirming established cases of tuberculosis it could screen patients with comparatively slight symptoms and act as the point at which apparently healthy persons who had been in close association with a tuberculous patient could be assembled and examined. The dispensary was a clearing house and a centre for observation from which patients could be directed to the most suitable place, home, hospital or sanatorium. Finally, the dispensary was also a treatment centre for ill patients: a point at which treatment was administered and from which treatment was monitored. In effect, the dispensary was 'the centre from which the manifold activities which safeguard the life of the sick person may be expected to radiate, and a bureau of research, information and education'.[3]

An extended medical gaze

The dispensary, of course, was not a new means of delivering health care; dispensaries had existed for centuries as means of providing treatments and advice for the poor. Yet in its old form the dispensary was a single immobile point at which medical assistance could be obtained, whereas the new dispensary, as founded in Edinburgh, represented a much more radical arrangement.

The new dispensary was a building, but also a new perceptual structure – a new way of *seeing* illness which manifested itself in different ways.*

First, and most apparent, it was a new way of organising health care, of effecting its geographical distributions. Whereas the hospital and out-patient clinic had operated more or less within their own walls, the dispensary radiated out into the community. Illness was sought, identified and monitored by various techniques and agents in the community; the dispensary building was merely the coordinating centre.

The need to establish a community presence arose from the new distributions of illness. Traditional hospital medicine, which had emerged at the end of the eighteenth century, had defined illness in terms of specific pathological lesions located within the confines of the body and the medical gaze aimed to observe the map – through signs and symptoms – the course of the disease within the space of the body.[4]

The new gaze, however, identified disease in the spaces between people, in the interstices of relationships, in the social body itself. In this new conceptualisation pathology was not an essentially static phenomenon to be localised to a specific point, but was seen to travel throughout the social body, appearing only intermittently. There was therefore a need for an organisational structure which could both survey and constantly monitor the whole community. Hence, also, the emphasis on close scrutiny of details of patients' contacts and relationships, and the creation of a thorough record of family networks, friends and acquaintances through which to coordinate home-visits, checks and follow-ups.

In effect, the Dispensary involved a double mapping of locality and relationships. The disease was geographically pin-pointed in the community ('a red mark on a map for every case') – as it had been during the great epidemics of the nineteenth century – so that its patterns and movements could be observed and interpreted. Superimposed on this geographical outline was the map of the social body on which, through screening and observation of patient contacts, a network of social relationships could be plotted. Gradually, as surveillance of patient contacts increased, the

* Hereafter I use the term 'dispensary' to refer to the traditional building and 'Dispensary' to embrace this new way of construing illness.

medical gaze began to focus with greater intensity on the potentially ill: the healthy and the normal.

In part, the Dispensary represented the Panopticon writ large, a whole community 'traversed throughout by heirarchy, surveillance, observation, writing'.[5] In this respect the Dispensary, as the Panopticon, had as its ideal project the town in the grip of plague, sub-divided, analysed, monitored, supervised, presenting a utopia of efficient social management and organisation. Yet there was also, as Foucault points out, another method of exercising power over men, 'of controlling their relations, of separating out their dangerous mixtures'. This was to be found in the image of the leper who gave rise to rituals of exclusion and, instead of the subtleties of multiple partitions and organisation in depth of surveillance and control, a massive binary division between one set of people and another.

In the nineteenth century both modes of control, multiple partitioning and binary separation, coexisted. Binary separation in the form of the mad/sane and the ill/healthy had its basis in the normal/abnormal dichotomy which had emerged in the mid eighteenth century. Yet within this bisected space the mad and the ill were subjected to the more sophisticated analyses of disciplinary partitioning in which the abnormal were separated out by diagnostic category and subjected to the surveillance techniques of a panoptic apparatus. The Panopticon itself was a mechanism of discipline and could, in principle, have been fixed on normal, abnormal or whole populations. However, during the nineteenth century, panoptic power was reserved primarily for the analysis of abnormal groups, in part as an attempt to use its corrective features to reform deviant bodies.

The Dispensary was, on the one hand, an extension of the panoptic vision to a whole society; on the other hand, its principle difference was its denial of the rituals of separation and exclusion that had characterised the exercise of panoptic power. In that the Dispensary required the social body to be monitored, it extended its gaze over the normal person to establish early detection, to advise on appropriate behaviour and relationships and to enable the potentially abnormal to be adequately known.

The domain of panopticism was 'that region of irregular bodies, with their details, their multiple movements, their heterogeneous forces, their spatial relations'; it required 'mechanisms that analyse distributions, gaps, series, combinations, and which use instruments that render visible, record, differentiate and compare: a physics of a relational and multiple power, which has its maximum intensity not in the person of the king, but in the bodies that can be individualised by their relations'.[6] The Dispensary further refined this gaze, these techniques of analysis, to fix them, not on individual bodies so much as the interstices of society; the Dispensary was a mechanism of power which imposed on the spatial arrangement of bodies the social configuration of their relationships. The Dispensary was a device, above all else, for making visible to constant surveillance the interaction between people, normal and abnormal, and thereby transforming the physical space between bodies into a social space traversed by power. At the beginning of the twentieth century the 'social' was born as an autonomous realm.[7]

Social hygiene

Power assumes a relationship based on some knowledge which creates and sustains it; conversely, power establishes a particular regime of truth in which certain knowledges become admissible or possible. The configuration of power to be found in the Dispensary was both a product of knowledge and the basis for a cognitive transformation of certain aspects of medicine in the early twentieth century.

Health was no longer to be regarded as a private and immutable state of a body, 'an inborn secret between the individual and his doctor', as Williams argued, but as something social and relative, 'an objective to which the individual could strive'.[8] The old regime treated the body as an object and attempted to control its relationship to the natural environment by identifying particular aetiological factors and promulgating sanitary laws of health which governed its activities. Hope's *Textbook of public health*, of 1915, perhaps typified the focus of attention by dealing with the dangers of site, soil, water, air and food.[9] With the advent of the social, the old 'public' health all but disappeared. As Hill pointed out in 1916: 'The old public health was concerned with the environment; the new is concerned with the individual'.[10] Within several decades new concerns intruded into the texts of public health. Burn's *Recent advances in public health*, of 1947, for example, contained a large section on 'public health and the individual' in which there was separate discussion of mother and child, nursery care, the school health service, health education, mental health services, dental health, medico–social services, the handicapped child, care of the family and welfare of the aged.[11]

Under the old system the natural environment was the potential source of ill-health. Under the new hygiene the natural environment was not of itself dangerous, but merely acted as a reservoir. The danger now arose from people and their points of contact. It was people who carried ill-health from the natural world into the social body and transmitted it within. The epidemiological gaze therefore began to shift from the environment to the mode of transmission between people and to ramifications of social relationships: 'Modern writers fail to find any useful or basic significance in contagions as contrasted with infections.'[12] The new hygiene, as proposed by Newman, depended on an educated people 'willing and able to practice the way of health'.[13] Preventive medicine was therefore no longer restricted to environmental questions and sanitation[14] but became concerned with the minutiae of social life. Might not health, Newman argued, be promoted 'by maintaining a clean mouth and clear breathing, and by abstinence from spitting, sneezing, coughing and shouting at each other?'[15]

The clinical gaze within the hospital had outlined and sustained the passive and discrete body by localising illnesses within it. In similar fashion the Dispensary gaze established the reality of the social by identifying diseases of social spaces, of contacts and relationships. Thus, as the social basis of the disease justified the Dispensary as the appropriate mechanism to combat it, so too the Dispensary established, by its deployment in the community, the social origins and character of the new health dangers.

Tuberculosis, which had, until the closing decades of the nineteenth century, been primarily a disease of individual bodies and of environmental neglect, became a disease of contact and social space. The techniques for monitoring the social can be seen in the increasing number of tuberculosis dispensaries established in the early decades of the twentieth century. They can be identified in the 'pilgrimage exhibitions' of the National Tuberculosis Association (founded 1898) to spread the dangers of casual social contact, which, by 1914, had distributed some 80 000 leaflets and books extolling the virtues of alertness to this disease of human mixings.[16] How better to keep the problem under constant surveillance than by pressing, from 1913 onwards, for the disease to be compulsorily notifiable? And from 1936, following the legal requirement for confidential registers of notified persons in 1930, to keep all contacts under observation for four years?[17]

Together, these various measures outlined a mechanism for social surveillance and for raising consciousness in the community thus observed. This greater consciousness, on the one hand enabled the intrusion of surveillance to be more easily justified, and, on the other hand made the potential patient a part of the surveillance mechanism. 'Intelligent individuals, realising their duty to their life partners and society at large' were therefore expected to consult their doctor on the social implications of their disease – Should they get married? Should they have children? Should they see their spouse?[18] Tuberculosis became a disease of human contact which, when adequately monitored, potentially revealed the social fabric of a community to an observing gaze.

The gaze of the Dispensary identified and constructed a social and sanitised area between individuals by the single device of using the knowledge that tuberculosis could be transmitted through 'respiratory contact'. The space between mouths and between noses became subjected to medical surveillance and the relationships, both familial and casual, which brought people into contact, became an item of medical record. It was the movement of the tuberculosis bacillus, invisible yet deadly, which outlined the social space between individuals.

For the purposes of a medical gaze, intent on focusing on the relationship between individuals, any disease such as tuberculosis which could be directly transmitted between people served to map social space. Thus the national outcry against the spread of venereal diseases early in the century was not only a manifestation of moral outrage but also of latent surveillance possibilities: the path of venereal diseases throughout the community traced the threads which linked one person intimately with another. The dangers of venereal disease could be used as a means of observing behaviour, educating thoughts and teaching contacts.

The Royal Commission, established in 1913 to investigate the whole problem of venereal disease, recommended a national system of 'clinics' to provide free diagnosis and an early campaign to educate the public.[19] The propaganda campaign was organised by the National Council for Combating Venereal Diseases, but it took the form of warnings against the dangers of illicit sexual encounters and a deliberate policy of avoiding advice on appropriate prophylactic measures subsequent to such an encounter, even though 'prophylactic packets' against venereal disease were available and had been used successfully in the army. These were not thought appropriate for civilians, however, as they could provide an incentive to immorality through removal of the fear of venereal disease. They would also, it was held, outrage public feeling and constitute a blow to a national crusade for higher standards of conduct.[20]

Yet the promulgation of these tactics of repression had a negative effect on the efficiency of the Dispensary. Free clinics were provided by local authorities but they remained stigmatised; compulsory notification was proposed but at the same time felt to be impractical in that it might drive the disease underground; and the tracing of contacts in the community could not proceed while fear governed the manifestations of the disease. This 'conspiracy of silence' which extended to even a mention of the diseases (did not syphilis and gonorrhoea 'sound evilly to the ear'[21]) prevented the Dispensary laying its observing networks on the threatened community and opening the secret and intimate movement of sexual contact to the meticulous hygiene of the medical gaze.

By the 1920s there was a noticeable shift in the emphasis of venereal disease propaganda. The moral connotations were less overtly stressed and the positive effects of combating the disease emerged. The emphasis of the work of the National Council was changed from fear to 'constructive' propaganda and a new name, The British Social Hygiene Council, was taken in 1925.[22] In 1930 the annual conference of the Council proposed increased provision for the treatment of venereal diseases and reported good follow-up of cases in Swansea.[23] Imperial social hygiene congresses were arranged to bring to the nation's attention the economic importance of combating venereal disease in the colonies: 'virility and efficiency of native races is of prime importance to the development of Empire'.[24] Through the techniques of social hygiene, venereal disease became a device for integrating a notion of illness – far removed from the closed world of the discrete body – with a system of civil administration, for there was now 'a general acceptance in every outpost of Empire that health and government were linked'.[25]

Venereal disease changed from being used as a means of forbidding certain relationships to a mechanism for observing them. The underlying social relationships themselves were brought into open discourse. The British Social Hygiene Council, instead of simply condemning illicit non-marital relationships, began to emphasise the need to 'promote social progress and preserve and strengthen the family'.[26] It produced a booklet on marriage, in 1932,[27] held a summer school of 'problems relating to family stability and preparation for marriage', in 1934[28] and produced a Year Book, in 1935, covering 'marine welfare, housing, maternity and child welfare, illegitimacy, juvenile delinquency, probation, deafness, and tuberculosis'.[29] The form of the Dispensary thereby fixed itself on the field of venereology and began to create a network of surveillance that monitored the social contacts, values and environment of recorded patients.

The child as object and problem

The technology of social hygiene which had, through the new contact diseases, established the identity of that invisible and problematic space between bodies, also manifested itself in the invention of the child as an object of the medical gaze. The body of the child was, of course, not only fabricated by the medical discourse that began to fix on it towards the end of the nineteenth century, but also by the various moral and educational concerns which contemporaneously enveloped it. At the same time as the body of every child was subjected to educational surveillance through the introduction of compulsory education the child entered medical discourse as a discrete object with attendant pathologies. Goodhart published the first edition of his *The diseases of children*, in 1885;[30] Hutchinson, his *Lectures on diseases of children*, in 1904;[31] and Garrod, his *Diseases of children*, in 1913.[32] A Society for the Study of Diseases in Children was founded in 1900 and in 1908 it became a founding Section of the Royal Society of Medicine.[33]

The figure of the child became caught up in a panoptic vision. Childhood was a state in which the child could be manipulated and transformed within the new field of observation established by the large halls of the new schools and the open wards of the new childrens' hospitals. As Cameron noted in his classic text, *The nervous child*, first published in 1919, 'the body of the child is moulded and shaped by the environment in which he grows. Pure air, a rational diet and free movement give strength and symmetry to every part.'[34]

However, while the figure of the child became caught up in a panoptic vision at the beginning of the twentieth century, it was also apparent that the child could not be adequately observed in isolation. The hospital, the clinic, the school were all admirable places from which to exercise surveillance over the child, yet they were not points from which the child could be observed in its 'natural' environment, namely, the home. Thus two related strategies can be identified as being developed around the child at the beginning of the century. First, there was the panoptic gaze which sought in the schools and hospitals to examine and inspect the actual body of the child; second, there was the Dispensary which attempted to map and survey the social relationships of the child in the community proper. It was Cameron's view that childhood should become part of the remit of preventive medicine: 'more and more a considerable part of the profession must busy itself in nurseries and schools, seeking to apply there the teachings of Psychology, Physiology, Heredity and Hygiene'.[35]

As these surveillance mechanisms increased in generality and intensity in the twentieth century, so too the apparent dangers from inadequately supervised children increased. Nervous children, delicate children, neuropathic children, maladjusted children, difficult children, over-sensitive children and unstable children were all essentially inventions of a new way of seeing childhood. 'A tendency to quarrel, to make violent friendships, to engender bitter dislikes, to attend unduly to bodily functions, to night terrors, to unreasonable fears, grief, introspection and self-examination and to separation from family and friends', marked out these potentially dangerous currents, dangerous because some of these children might 'eventually rise to a high career in public affairs'.[36]

Milk depots were opened in various towns in the early years of the twentieth century to provide milk (bottled under hygienic conditions) to mothers with small babies. Attendance at a milk depot meant that the children were closely scrutinised: they were weighed once a week, their homes were visited by health visitors who reported their progress to the Medical Officer of Health and the mothers were provided with cards on which to record the weight of their child. While on the one hand the milk depots praised the value of breast milk, in their practice they encouraged attendance to obtain cow's milk so that the child could come under observation. In effect, the milk depot functioned as a surveillance apparatus, integrating in a hierarchy of observation the Medical Officer of Health, health visitor and mother and compiling for the body of each young child an individual dossier.[37]

But what of the mothers who declined to bring their children to the milk depots? How could the gaze extend itself to this child who was unknown to the medical services? This problem had been tackled in Huddersfield in 1905 by paying the mother one shilling for notifying the birth within 24 hours to the MOH. This scheme of birth notification was made compulsory in 1906 for Huddersfield, and in 1907 a National Birth Notification Act was passed, in 1915 becoming compulsory. With notification of births, visits from assistant MOsH, constant observation by the health visitor and the requirement, from 1910, that only qualified midwives and doctors could supervise the actual birth, the child, from its very moment of entry into the world, became an object of medical interest, for the first time a visible body with its own individual record.

A national campaign against infant mortality was established on the basis, as McCleary has observed, that deaths in the first year of life were not a problem of sanitation so much as of personal hygiene.[38] Maternity benefit was introduced – available to those mothers who registered the impending birth – and ante-natal clinics were founded. Baby clinics, day nurseries and nursery schools were opened, each establishing a point from which to observe the behaviour and relationships of the young child.

Medical surveillance of the older child was entrusted to the school medical service which was established in 1908 following the report of the 1904 Interdepartmental Committee on Physical Deterioration.[39] The service was provided through two clinics, one for treatment and one for inspection. The treatment clinic operated as a panoptic structure: a point at which bodies were individually examined, abnormalities diagnosed and appropriate treatment provided. The inspection clinic, on the other hand, followed the structure of the Dispensary. It screened all school children at varying times for incipient and manifest disease; it organised visits to childrens' homes by the school nurse to report on conditions, monitor progress and advise mothers on the care and treatment of their children. And it functioned as a co-ordination centre: records of children were maintained, reports from the community were filed, observations were up-dated. 'From it [the inspection clinic] should be directed and organised the work of the School Medical Officer, school nurse, attendance officer and Care Committee.'[40]

It was at the beginning of the twentieth century, therefore, that a link was forged between systems of educational and medical surveillance. On the one hand, the educational system provided a mechanism for one component of the Dispensary: the inculcation of social hygiene. Hygiene was 'an integral part of the ordinary school routine ... a practice rather than a theory, a way of life rather than an abstract idea'.[41] On the other hand, the medical system provided a mechanism to monitor educational progress. Inspection clinics became assessment as well as diagnostic centres, in part to offer, within a medical discourse, reasons for educational failure. With the later growth of child guidance and the localisation of the vagaries of mental development to the innocence of childhood, a parallel school psychological service emerged to focus on the latent mind of the child.

Social space and social time

The Dispensary offered a reconstruction of social space and of social time. Where panopticism had, in effect, offered to the observing eye that which was in an enclosed space, the school, the hospital or the prison, the Dispensary, through its juxtaposition of observation and community, replaced enclosed physical space with an open and social domain.

A focus on space – in buildings and between bodies – was not new to the medical world of the twentieth century. The sanatorium for tuberculosis, with its emphasis on open air, had originated in 1840 when Bodington recommended 'a pure atmosphere, freely demonstrated without fear'.[42] The growth of sanatoria, however, was slow, especially in England, until the closing decade of the nineteenth century and it was not until the early twentieth century that the space surrounding and between bodies came into sharper medical focus. Nineteenth-century miasmatic theory, which had stressed the dangers of impure air, was – in a new form – revived in the claim that pure air was beneficial to health.

The once dark and enclosed school was opened up: large windows which could be opened during lessons to allow the passage of air were recommended. School hygiene was discussed in public health textbooks in terms of a school design which would allow free space to circulate around the child.[43] The first open-air school was opened in 1907 by the London County Council and by 1931 there were 80 such schools catering for 9000 children.[44] Even in schools with traditional architecture it was recommended that classes be held outside, in the yard or in the park. The *Lancet*, in supporting this policy, suggested that on cold days exercises could be given at regular intervals to keep the children warm.[45]

The outdoor conditions were intimately bound up with the new conception of health. They were not intended for the fittest students but, on the contrary, for the relatively unfit. Spartan conditions had been a system for strengthening already strong bodies but in the Dispensary they were deployed around the weakest. Open-air schools were recommended for 'debilitated, undernourished children, those with incipient pulmonary tuberculosis and children who were nervous and excitable'. It became official policy to admit more and more nervous and maladjusted children to these open schools.[46]

Industrial efficiency was studied in the context of air, temperature, humidity, movement. Air conditioning and ventilation were discussed jointly by hygienists and clinicians.[47] The old idea of closed wards and mechanical ventilation to prevent the transmission of microbes was reversed and 'natural cross ventilation' recommended.[48] Though at first only used on the tuberculous patient, such ideas became equally applicable to medical, surgical and infectious-disease wards and in convalescent homes. Hygienic space itself became therapeutic, open windows (together with warmer clothing) could promote health.[49]

The construction and management of space within hospitals was no longer simply governed by panoptic principles through which all detail might be visible – but by notions of a hygienic and social matrix in which bodies mixed. 'Have we yet designed the ideal ward block? What are the proper amounts of wall space and floor space for patients of different types?'[50] Even in the siting of such hospitals it was advised to use the 'health-giving' factors of a site to their maximum advantage.[51]

The new hygiene opened up the space around bodies just as purposefully as it had opened up the space around the hospital or clinic. The Dispensary offered a perceptual structure which operated in an open yet essentially social space. It offered an analysis of bodies in space – a space through which bodies met and interaction took place. The old system of quarantine excluded, the new system allowed a controlled passage. 'Quarantine is the source of all our preventive method against the spread of infectious disease . . . The dominating principle of modern as opposed to the old quarantine is that it must be a sieve not a dam.'[52]

The conceptualisation of space in which the Dispensary operated – in the community and around bodies – could also be found in the cognitive spatialisation of the new diseases. Panopticism had been a reductionist gaze, sub-dividing space in the hospital and in the body. Pathology was localised and static. The Dispensary, on the other hand, revived an older tradition from the eighteenth century, before tissue pathology came to dominate clinical medicine, when disease existed within the body but manifested itself without regularity at one point, then later at another. Symptoms appeared, disappeared, reappeared. The symptoms in this old regime could no more be used to localise a pathology than could actual physical examination of the body. Symptoms constituted a somewhat random manifestation of the illness through bodily space and time and the physician's task was simply to wait, to observe and to listen.[53]

Similarly, the Dispensary did not localise pathology. A single patient with venereal disease was simply a manifestation of a disease which in all probability had already moved on and was manifesting itself elsewhere. Venereal disease might disappear from a patient but re-emerge in a casual acquaintance, then later reappear in the original patient. Disease was constituted in the social body and it was the social movement of the disease, as it traversed that body, which had to be observed, monitored and interpreted, thereby establishing by its analysis the very existence of that same social space. Whereas the clinical gaze that was established at the end of the eighteenth century made, for the first time, the space of disease coterminous with the space of the body,[54] the extended gaze of the twentieth century discovered in the new diseases a pathological form which was superimposed on the outline of the social body.

Where the Panopticon was a device for monitoring and constituting bodies, the Dispensary was a mechanism for surveying, and thereby rendering problematic, particular relationships between those same bodies. In its institutional arrangements – the tuberculosis dispensary, the venereal disease clinic, the school medical service inspection clinic or the child welfare clinic – the Dispensary cast an observing eye over the community. Counting, assessing, tracing, following, recording, coordinating, the Dispensary constructed the outlines of a social map in which particular social relationships came into increasing focus through their constant and meticulous scrutiny. At the same time both justification and explanation were provided for this surveillance by the 'invention' of new medical problems – venereal diseases, tuberculosis, the nervous child, infant mortality, the feckless mother – which, if left unsupervised, might have threatened the very fabric of society, but which, when adequately monitored, could serve instead to throw into relief the essential social bonds that linked one person with another.

In 1912 the Section of Epidemiology of the Royal Society of Medicine (one of its founder sections) extended its purposes: to observe the *persistence*, as well as the variability, of disease in the community.[55] The new medicine had to address itself to time, to the movement of pathology rather than its localisation.

3

Invention of the neuroses

In 1906 Bruce published his *Studies of clinical psychiatry* – a standard textbook of psychiatry which dealt exclusively with the classification, aetiology, diagnosis and treatment of insanity.[1] In 1944, the sixth edition of Henderson and Gillespie's *A textbook of psychiatry* was offering considerable space to the 'psychoneuroses' and, moreover, had decided to place them before discussion of the 'psychoses' (the new term for insanity) 'because they are much more common'.[2] How was it that within the space of less than 40 years the object of psychiatric interest had changed so much? How had the psychoneuroses emerged into such prominence? And how had insanity (or madness) suffered a change and relative decline in importance?

Insanity and neurasthenia

The problem of madness had first come into prominence some two centuries earlier, in the Age of Reason. Foucault has argued that the moment of its discovery, when Pinel struck off the chains of the madmen in Bicêtre, did not, however, signify a new liberation as much as the full institutionalisation and confinement of madness.[3] With its new classification, madness was separated from debauchery, criminality, idleness, vagabondage and vagrancy (to all of which it had seemed as one) and confined to the asylum: 'The obscure guilt that once linked transgression and unreason is thus shifted; the madman, as a human being originally endowed with reason, is no longer guilty of being mad.'[4] As a result, madness became imprisoned in a 'moral world' which successfully delineated the world of reason from unreason.[5] Confinement protected the pure community and sanity was reaffirmed by the exile of the insane.[6]

Towards the end of the nineteenth century a new problem of mental functioning began to emerge. It was observed that some people suffered from 'mental instability' which did not of itself constitute madness; medical attention started to focus, not on unreason, but on the vagaries of apparently ordinary mental functioning. Undoubtedly, other diagnostic categories – cholorosis, anaemia, even malingering – had been used previously to classify problems of mental instability;[7] but in these diagnoses, nervous irritability had represented only one (and perhaps a minor) manifestation of the condition. Mental instability began to be defined as a problem in its own right only towards the end of the nineteenth century when the neuroses were constituted as objects of medical discourse.[8]

One of the earliest manifestations of the new problem of mental instability can be found in the diagnoses of 'nerves' and 'neurasthenia'. In the first two decades of the twentieth century, neurasthenia took its place in medical textbooks, together with hysteria and psychasthenia, as the most important of the so-called neuroses. Neurasthenia was variously described but it seemed to be mainly characterised by nerve 'exhaustion' or fatigue.[9] It was believed to be brought about by over-exertion, and treatment was mainly by rest and routine.

Psychiatry, the specialty of the insane, incorporated these manifestations of mental instability into its theories of madness by describing them as precursors of insanity. The neuroses were simply symptoms or early warnings of impending madness. In his textbook *Psychological medicine*, of 1905, Craig sub-divided his chapter on general neuroses into three sections: epilepsy and insanity, hysteria and insanity, and traumatic neuroses.[10] Cole, too, in his *Mental diseases*, published in 1913, classified the neuroses under the heading 'neuroses and insanity' – a classification which continued up to the third edition of the book published in 1924.[11]

The brevity of the discussion of the neuroses and their treatment as precursors of insanity, to be found in these psychiatric texts, can partly be explained by the fact that psychiatrists claimed rarely to see the condition. As Craig & Beaton pointed out in 1926, 'until quite recently the neurologists never saw the case of insanity shut up in the mental hospitals and the mental hospital physician, the alienists or psychiatrists never saw the case of "nerves"'.[12] It was therefore left to the neurologist, the general physician and the general practitioner to cope with these 'new' complaints. In consequence, neurasthenia appeared contemporaneously in the neurological textbooks as primarily a neurological problem. Although it might manifest itself as an affliction of the mind, as 'nerves', fatigue or 'brain fag', its basis, it was claimed, was decidedly neurological.[13] And as disease was 'inconceivable without some underlying physical basis'[14], functional disorders such as neurasthenia, in which there was apparently tissue 'dysfunction' [*sic*] without structural abnormality, were seen to be rooted in real if unrecognised physical processes.[15]

Medicalisation of the mind

The uneasy relationship between the old disease of madness and the new problem of the neuroses in psychiatry was transformed in the second decade of the new century. The change is shown, somewhat dramatically, in the third edition of Stoddart's textbook, *Mind and its disorders.*[16] The previous editions had devoted the customary chapter to neurasthenia – an illness characterised by mental fatigue – which might be bestowed on their progeny by parents who had used up their stock of nervous energy. The third edition of 1919, however, reported that 'since the last edition I have fundamentally changed my attitude towards mental disease'.[17] Stoddart confessed to having been influenced by the new Freudian ideas: he now included a chapter on psychoanalysis, introduced the notion of anxiety neurosis and, following Freud, suggested that neurasthenia was a product of auto-eroticism and masturbation.

Many of Stoddart's psychiatric colleagues, however, were less enthusiastic about the new ideas. The second edition of Cole's textbook, published in the same year, found 'food for reflection' in the psychoneuroses[18] but only added anxiety neurosis as a diagnostic category in the third edition of 1924. Norman's textbook of 1928, *Mental disorders for students and practitioners,* continued to link all mental disorders to insanity and gave only one mention of the Freudian school, while remarking: 'there seems some difference of opinion in this respect'.[19] Devine's book of 1929, on *Recent advances in psychiatry,* dealt exclusively with the psychoses (the new term for the insane).[20] Cannon & Hayes in their textbook of 1932, *The principles and practice of psychiatry,* acknowledged anxiety and neuroses as psychogenic problems but only in as much as they might contribute towards insanity.[21]

If Stoddart was an exception to the general trend it is perhaps worth noting that in 1919 he was no longer a mental hospital superintendent; when he was 'converted' to Freudian psychopathology he was a lecturer in mental diseases at St Thomas's Hospital Medical School. In moving from the world of the asylum to the general hospital he reflected the difference in attitudes towards mental disease in these two domains. During the 1920s and 1930s the main thrust for the incorporation of problems of mental instability (and of Freudian ideas) into medicine came, not from a psychiatry rooted in the asylum, but from a general medicine faced with a generalised problem of mental functioning.

While psychiatric textbooks tended to ignore the new developments these latter were rapidly taken up by neurologists[22] and found their way into the neurological texts. Stewart, the author of *The diagnosis of nervous disease,* had completely rewritten the chapter on psychoneuroses in the sixth edition of 1924. While he still felt that these mental diseases manifested themselves through 'molecular changes' the new terminology of conscious, unconscious, complexes, etc., was explained.[23] Similarly, Thompson's *Diseases of the nervous system*, of 1915 (second edition), accepted that neurasthenia merged into anxiety neurosis and by 1921 (third edition) used the familiar Freudian language in which to describe mental pathology.[24]

The appearance of the psychoneuroses in medical texts formalised an increasing concern of general medicine with the mind. The mind in all its detail had become important – not the diseased mind of the mad or insane, but the ordinary mind of everyone. As Sir Humphrey Rolleston, Regius Professor of Physic at Cambridge and President of the Royal College of Physicians, claimed in 1925: 'probably the bulk of patients in ordinary practice present some disorder, however slight, of mind, conduct or feeling'.[25]

The diagnosis of insanity had been a ritual of exclusion; the madman, like the leper, was caught up in a regime of rejection and exile. Within the confinement of the asylum, it is true, there had been a panoptic gaze which sought to observe, analyse and partition the amorphous mass of the insane, but these techniques were only secondary to the great binary division of madness from sanity which informed the psychiatric method. Madness represented the political dream of a pure community by marking the mad. In contrast, the neuroses celebrated the ideal of a disciplined society in which all were analysed and distributed.

Neurasthenia had enabled the identification of the fatigued and exhausted; the neuroses recognised stress and its effects. At first, while neurasthenia still survived, it was the stress of masturbation; later it became more generalised – a medical eye on stresses of childhood, parenting, workshops, schools and homes. Those forces, ever present in social space, which impinged on the functioning of individual bodies, were theoretically refined into a discourse on stress and coping. A general medicine which, since the beginning of the nineteenth century, had offered surveillance and examination of the deviant body, extended its 'gaze' to the mind of everyone.

The deployment of this new medical gaze to the mind of everyone involved various tactics. First its limitless range was affirmed. Neurasthenia, which tended to be inherited by the few, gradually disappeared to be replaced by the neuroses, which might appear in anyone. Neurasthenia was reputedly in decline during the 1920s[26] and it was left to Buzzard, the king's physician and Regius Professor of Medicine at Oxford, to declare it merely a 'dumping ground' for inadequately recognised cases of anxiety neurosis and depression.[27]

Second, the deployment of a medical gaze over the mind inevitably brought conflict with those bodies and institutions which had traditionally kept a guard over certain specific aspects of mental functioning. In an address in 1927, entitled 'Medicine and the church', Buzzard warned the clergy against interfering in the treatment of the mind. It was, he claimed, the 'one bone of contention' between church and medicine. 'I have taken the courage of my profession in my two hands today and have declared that we make no claim to spiritual healing.... Any fears I may entertain are for the Church, who if she listens to some of her disciples, might find herself in competition, not with medicine, but with quacks and charlatans.'[28]

The other group whose unorganised activities threatened the unified medical gaze were lay people who practised psychotherapy. Ross claimed in his Morison Lectures of 1935 that there were grave dangers in allowing unqualified lay people to treat mental disorders.[29] These dangers, the *Lancet* suggested, lay in the fact that physical and mental illness could not be sharply separated so the psychotherapist must of necessity have a basic training in the rest of medicine.[30]

Third, if the new medical gaze to the mind was to be effective then it would have to be adequately taught. In its annual review of medical education, in 1920, the *British Medical Journal* made its usual perfunctory mention of psychological medicine: 'The study of mental disorders has long been a necessary part of the ordinary medical curriculum.'[31] In 1921 it added the qualification that it had also been 'somewhat neglected'.[32] In 1922, it had both been neglected and 'its importance scarcely recognised.... Of late it has become apparent that mental disorder constitutes a social and medical problem of great significance, and there is little doubt that in future it will be recognised as one of the most important specialities.' This newly important aspect of medicine was no longer constrained to the severe forms in the asylum but included 'mild and often unrecognised psychoses and various types of psychoneuroses'.[33]

Bernard Hart, in 1918, had first proposed that psychology be taught in the medical curriculum and George Newman, the Chief Medical Officer, had also commended it in a memorandum to the Ministry of Health in 1923.[34] The British Association was sufficiently concerned to appoint a committee to consider the place of 'normal psychology' in the medical curriculum. It reported in 1928 that in half the country's medical schools there was no instruction in this area.[35] The *Lancet* thought this 'absurdly inadequate' given that psychological medicine was no longer confined to the asylum but embraced 'a far wider field'.[36] *The British Medical Journal* agreed that normal (and abnormal) psychology was a necessary part of any medical curriculum: 'it is now universally admitted that a large part of every doctor's practice consists of minor conditions of a "functional" nature'.[37]

Debates ensued about the type of psychology which should be taught and about whether it should be taught by psychiatrists, physicians or surgeons;[38] but, as the *Lancet* pointed out, the issue of whether more instruction was desirable was not in dispute.[39] Psychology had become an indispensable part of medicine and this position would have to be reflected in the curriculum.

Fourth, the new medical gaze to the mind of everyone was also an examination of the mind of the individual. Yet that individual was not a 'given' but had itself been fabricated as a physical object within the older medical gaze of the panoptic vision. The new regime therefore called for an integrated gaze, a synthesis of the physical and the psychological, so that the individual, both organically and mentally, could be subjected to a single analysis.

On the one hand, this unitary gaze could be effected by treating the physical and the psychological as two sides of the same coin. The Royal Commission on Lunacy and Mental Disorder, which reported in 1926, argued: 'There is no clear line of demarcation between mental and physical illness ... a mental illness may have physical concomitants ... a physical illness may have, and probably always has, mental concomitants.'[40] On the other hand, there were various attempts in the inter-war years to construct a 'unified theory' of mind–body relations. Pavlov's experiments in conditioned reflexes, reported in his 1928 Croonian Lecture, was research, the *Lancet* felt, which belonged to the borderland of physiology and psychology;[41] Meyer proposed the notion of reaction-types to explain biological reactivity to psychological stimuli;[42] Adler argued that mental tension manifested itself in defective organs and endocrine inbalance.[43]

The belief in the 'indissoluble unity of mind and body' was the basis for membership of the Medical Society of Individual Psychology, founded in 1931. Its chairman, Langdon-Brown, the Regius Professor at Cambridge, confessed that 'sheer force of experience' had led him 'to realise the need for a more psychological approach to medicine ... as many people were ill because they were unhappy, as were unhappy because they were ill'.[44] He, personally, felt that the sympathetic nervous system – especially the pituitary – was of misunderstood importance in the genesis of mental disorder.[45] Other members of the Society suggested that there were problems of 'fine adjustment of organic senses in psychoneurotics, in particular poor sight and wax in the ears', or there was a problem of 'tight collars and tight shoes', or that 'hyperthyroidism, septic tonsils, constipation and oxalicia' were to blame. Little sympathy was offered to the one-sided theories, derived from Freud and Jung, which were imbued with 'a great deal of washy and spineless eclecticism that degenerates into clinical opportunism, if not humbug'.[46]

The Tavistock Clinic, together with its associated Institute of Medical Psychology, also promoted a unified psychosomatic approach to diagnosis and treatment, and for most of the inter-wars years had to keep its waiting list closed, such was the demand for treatment.[47] Crichton-Miller, the Clinic's founder, published his views on aetiology in 1920 in his book, *Functional nerve disease.* There he argued that the emotions, sepsis, the endocrines and blood circulation, all had interdependent effects on mental stability.[48]

His approach was undoubtedly supported by the Medical Advisory Board of the Clinic, which included the physicians Buzzard and Langdon-Brown and the 'philosopher–surgeon', Trotter. Despite the Clinic's later reputation for promoting psychodynamic techniques, a detailed physical examination was carried out in almost every case for specific organic lesions such as focal sepsis or thyroid disfunction.[49]

This approach was maintained by Crichton-Miller's successor, Rees, who, in a textbook on psychological medicine, published in 1936, continued to argue that anxiety symptoms were caused by sympathetic and para-sympathetic nerve function. Surely, he argued, 'there must be a direct connection between physiology of the nervous system and psychology' such that there is a 'vicious circle of mental and physical inter-action'.[50] Had not the Freudian dream once been the rooting of mental functioning in cerebral physiology?

It would be misleading, however, to suggest that there was a broad consensus on theories of mental disorder; there was certainly a struggle between, for example, the exclusively psychogenic British Psychoanalytic Society and the notion of psychosomatic unity so strong in general medicine. Yet it would be equally inappropriate to characterise the debate simply as one between psychodynamic and organic theories. The struggle lay, not between theories, but within the myriad interactions that occurred daily between a gaze and its object, a disciplined mind.

The mind was represented to the gaze in words. Whereas under the old regime the body of the patient had to be made legible to the physician's interrogation, under the new regime the body produced its own truth which required, not legibility, but encouragement. The patient had to speak, to confess, to reveal; illness was transformed from what was visible to what was heard. The social space between doctor and patient became, not an impediment to the legibility of the passive body, but the complex matrix in which words were captured and the mind crystallised.

It would be wrong to say the mind was discovered, as that presumes it had an existence prior to the gaze; but neither could it be said to have independent existence after its fabrication other than in the discourse, strategies and interaction that gave it meaning. As in the analysis of the social, it is necessary to be nominalist. The social was created by a gaze which relentlessly mapped and monitored the physical space between bodies and it is in this same space that the mind was constituted. In the nineteenth century the mind had been a faculty of rationality coterminous with the cerebral tissues; in the twentieth century the mind was established in a social space of relationships and interaction which, according to contemporary theories, were both of causal significance, and particular manifestations by which it might be observed. This is not to imply that these contemporary theories were anything but links, in terms of the new regime of truth, between the various elements of mental disorder which emerged at the beginning of the century. Equally, the institutional settings, professional structures and organisational settings which developed around the mind, were both phenomena that sustained the existence of the mind and, at the same time, products of the monitored space between bodies in which the mind and the social were born.

The mind, as it was observed in the inter-war years, was therefore a fabrication of the disciplinary mechanisms of the Dispensary. The medical gaze shifted from body to mind: a focus on relationships and on interaction; a conceptualisation of pathology as existing in the social body, constantly appearing, disappearing, reappearing; a need to know of its various manifestations and the development of techniques for its observation; a gaze turned on the 'normal' population, as much as on the diseased, in an attempt to identify the incipient signs of instability; a medicine focused, not on the mind of the mad, but on the mind of the precariously sane. Insanity and neurasthenia had been afflictions of those constitutionally predisposed; neurosis was a potential problem for everyone. As Ross argued in his book on *The common neuroses*, in 1923, the difficulties experienced by the neurotic were greater by far for him than they were for normal people 'but they are the same difficulties which all of us have'.[51]

A perpetual gaze

Rolleston, in arguing that the bulk of patients in ordinary practice had disorder of mind, conduct or feeling, also charged that 'the earlier departures from the normal should be communicated to the doctor and remedial measures started without delay'.[52] A medicine which gazed into the smallest interstices of human lives could maintain an orderly society. A constant surveillance over mental functioning could keep at bay the manifestations of stress which threatened the precarious strands that made up the social order.

The observation and surveillance of the mind started with the child. The advantage of dealing with the child was the potential for change:

'[children's] abnormalities are as unshaped as their normalities and they can often be modelled to what shape we please'.[53] The child was father of the man. Moreover, 'children are not born with a highly developed faculty of control or sense of responsibility. They have to acquire our standards of right and wrong carefully, and in many cases with difficulty.' By the age of twelve or fourteen the correct instincts were normally present 'but in a certain number of people a tendency to dishonesty and untruthfulness persists into young adult life, and may die only with the person'.[54]

A strategy was therefore devised to guard against such unwanted outcomes. The GP could observe the child and advise on correct parenting.[55] Schools could monitor the progress of the child, not simply by examinations, but by such new techniques of surveillance as serial psychometric testing and through the new discipline of educational psychology.[56] The mental welfare of children could be secured by a new medicine of children[57] (British Paediatric Association, founded 1928), new clinics (Children's Clinic for the Treatment and Study of Nervous and Delicate Children, founded 1928), new research establishments[58] (National Institute of Child Psychology, founded 1931) and the notion of child guidance to correct, at an early stage, the potential instability of adult life (Child Guidance Council, founded 1927).[59]

The problems in the mental life which was provided for the child manifested themselves as new diagnostic groups. Cameron identified the nervous child as a product of parental neglect of proper mental development, in 1911;[60] the Sections of Psychiatry and of Diseases in Children at the Royal Society of Medicine jointly discussed the 'difficult child', in 1929[61], and the 'eneuretic child', in 1934[62]; in his chapter in *Diseases of children* Guthrie focused on the 'neurotic child';[63] the Chief Medical Officer at the Board of Education recognised the 'neuropathic child', in 1920, the 'maladjusted child', in 1927, and the 'unstable child', in 1928;[64] special educational provision was made for the 'delicate child' and the 'nervous child';[65] medical concern was expressed for the 'over-sensitive child' and for the 'solitary child'.[66] The child was construed as precariously normal, as liable to slip into inappropriate or problem behaviour without constant vigilance. The solitary child, for example, suffered from not being a child, from constant attempts to be like an adult when this was not appropriate behaviour. Moreover, like other problems of children, the problem of the solitary child was not restricted in its range of application to particular children. Any child could suffer from 'only childism' if not properly reared.[67]

All this, however, was not enough: 'Can we produce healthy babies until we have produced mentally secure parents? . . . Not until we have had one or two generations of infants brought up from birth to maturity in accordance with the best principles of mental hygiene.'[68] As early as 1919, Buzzard, in his Presidential Address to the Section of Psychiatry at the Royal Society of Medicine, advocated 'rational mental hygiene' and argued that it should be taught to medical students so that GPs would know of it.[69] Henderson, in his Morison Lectures for 1931, proposed that mental hygiene should be placed on the same footing as physical hygiene with centralised control vested in public health officials. Many forms of disordered conduct were believed due to an individual's inability to adapt himself to the demands of everyday life 'and a hopeful method of approach was to deal with those who had not yet developed any outstanding defect'.[70]

Moral education, social responsibility, healthy relationships and happy marriages would need to be engendered throughout the population. 'The sense of meaningful community must be re-created at a higher turn of the spiral.' Social class differences were outmoded, it was argued, and they needed to be replaced with insight based on friendly participation. 'This technique applies at all levels, in the home, in education, in industry and in politics and is essentially the same technique as that used in modern psychotherapy.'[71]

The strategy of mental hygiene could also be deployed in industry: behind industrial problems were to be found problems of mental functioning. In a study by the Industrial Fatigue Research Board, neuroses were found to underlie telegraphists' cramp.[72] Similarly, the organic lesion of miners' nystagmus was gradually construed as a neurotic one.[73] Industrial hygiene, the Chief Inspector of Factories advised, should be taught in schools and 'workers should be specially kept under observation during their first year' to see how 'accident-prone' they were.[74]

The value of this approach for industry had already been shown by studies in the USA by Mayo in the late 1920s and by the emergence of the 'human relations' school of factory management. In Britain too, the deployment of mental hygiene could increase industrial production, relieve boredom, give pride in work, improve morale, provide incentives, and so on.[75] Mental hygiene could enable the surveillance of everyone so the misfit could be identified: 'the socially inefficient, the unemployable, the epileptic, the habitual offender, the prostitute, and all others who have not been able to fit themselves harmoniously into the fabric of society'.[76]

The new perception over the mind of everyone was at once both a gaze over the community and a detailed study of the individual. The investigation of the individual, 'from every aspect, without reference to obsolete and misleading academic distinctions'[77], enabled the individual to be classified, graded and placed in his or her rightful place within the community. 'Once such a classification is made, a capable medical man is able by appropriate treatment, to raise many from lower to higher classes ... practical psychology, with medical co-operation, could also be used for the grading of young people into classes suitable for different kinds of work.'[78]

The Dispensary provided a new technology to ensure that 'square pegs are fitted into square holes'.[79] A system based on ascription or achievement could be replaced by one based on observation, tests, interviews, questionnaires, analyses, selection and follow-up. During World War II new recruits were physically examined for fitness, but it was felt that much more could be done to weed out the mentally unfit.[80] The new techniques of personnel selection were applied rigorously to the officer class and it was recommended that psychologists and psychiatrists could just as profitably be used in monitoring military and civilian appointments in peacetime.[81]

The adoption of this vision of mental health provided a means of controlling a population – without repression – through constant mapping and surveillance. But it did more than control: it reordered and restructured. Personality was 'corrected' by personality[82] and the potential threat to civilisation of latent mental disorder could be constantly counteracted. The school medical service and the prison medical service, for example, allowed the doctor to detect 'numerous higher-grade defectives, many of whom are a menace to the community by reason of their criminal propensities'.[83] GPs could 'have their fingers not only on the pulses of their individual patients but on the social pulse of the war-time community in which they live'.[84] From the teacher in the school and the psychiatric social worker in the community, right up to the suggested expert in psychological medicine in the Cabinet Office[85], a vast mechanism was proposed to monitor the mental well-being of the community at a time when every kind of mental disorder seemed to be on the increase.[86] A community was no longer conceived of as being fixed and immobile but as being flexible and malleable; it might be threatened by the very discussion of mental instability,[87] but if reconstituted it might possess undreamed of strengths.

A new psychological medicine

While general medicine showed increasing concern with psychological matters, such that medical psychology could show 'meteoric' growth,[88] mental hospital psychiatry remained basically opposed to psychodynamic ideas.[89] Nevertheless, changes in status and in the relationship of psychiatry to general medicine were signalled by the granting of the Royal prefix to the psychiatrists' professional organisation the Medico–Psychological Association in 1926. There were changes too in the perception of the mentally ill, signified by the Royal Commission and ensuing Mental Treatment Act of 1930 which abolished the term 'asylum' and replaced the term 'insanity' with 'of unsound mind'.

The perceptual structure which had excluded and isolated the insane had also functioned to separate off their attendant medical practitioners. A conjoining of the insane with other medical patients – either with milder mental disorder or with physical illness – could serve to legitimate a commensurate reunion of psychiatry with general medicine.

In 1926 Lord published his *The clinical study of mental disorder*, in which he claimed that 'unavoidable circumstances' in the form of legislation had kept psychiatry and general medicine apart. Now was the time for reintegration as there were fundamentally 'no sharp divisions between clinical psychiatry, clinical psychology and clinical neurology'. 'Psychiatry', he argued, 'should be wider than insanity.'[90]

In 1926 also, Craig published the fourth edition of his *Psychological medicine* (with a new co-author, Beaton). In this new edition the separation of psychiatric from other medical problems was decried: 'insanity is a separate conception with no real meaning in scientific medicine'. It was simply a legal rather than medical classification. Problems of behaviour and mental complaints had too long been separated – they were one continuum. In consequence, 'mental disorder is increasingly taking place as a branch of medical science, not to be divorced from but rather to be more closely linked with general medicine'.[91]

It was still possible, in the same text, to completely ignore Freudian explanations in a rewritten chapter on the 'psychoneuroses and the allied psychoses'. The validity of the Freudian doctrine, however – and the acrimonious discussion which surrounded it – was not the issue. The important point was that 'the insane patient is ill. He looks ill.'[92] Insanity was a medical problem. Moreover, this reinvigorated psychiatric medicine of the mind was not just the study of unreason: 'it means the study of the whole individual ... the patient must be regarded as a biological whole'.[93]

This new perception of the nature of mental illness was further inscribed in the new institutional arrangement which emerged to cope with the new epidemic. The long waiting list for treatment at the Tavistock Clinic in the inter-war years gave some indication of the iceberg of morbidity which had been revealed and which required out-patient services.[94] Moreover, the effect of providing adequate out-patient facilities had been demonstrated in the experimental liaison between the Littlemore Mental Hospital and the Radcliffe Infirmary in Oxford when the expansion of the out-patient department for nervous disorders at the Radcliffe had been matched by a corresponding decline in the population of the mental hospital.[95]

The policy of encouraging psychiatric out-patients departments in general hospitals was endorsed by the Royal Commission on Lunacy in

1926 and embodied in the Mental Treatment Act of 1930. The result was that more out-patients departments were established, sometimes attached to teaching or general hospitals, sometimes to mental hospitals. General and teaching hospitals established their own psychiatric beds[96] and appointed psychiatrists to their staffs (initially often in the department of neurology).[97] Psychiatric training also came to reflect the new divisions within the psychiatric task.[98]

If there is one gesture which can illustrate the sum effect of these changes in inter-war psychiatry it is in the different worlds of perception signified by the frontispiece of Cole's *Mental diseases*, which, from 1913 to 1924, showed a coloured picture of the diseased brain of general paralysis of the insane,[99] and the dedication of Henderson & Gillespie's *Textbook of psychiatry*, from 1927 to the present day, to the 'imaginative leadership' of Meyer.[100] In the former, the ideal of psychiatry was reduced to a simple pathological lesion, in the latter it was expanded into the meticulous study of individual 'reaction-types'. From that moment, the psychoses needed no longer to be excluded;[101] psychiatry could embrace 'variations ranging from gross madness to inconspicuous peculiarities of disposition'.[102] 'It is in this broader, more social, more biological conception that psychiatry today differs so greatly from its past.'[103]

4

A medicine of the social

In 1920 the Consultative Council on Medical and Allied Services of the Ministry of Health (chaired by Lord Dawson) published an *Interim report on the future provision of medical and allied services.*[1] In answer to the request by the Minister of Health to 'make recommendations as to the scheme or schemes requisite for the systematised provision of . . . medical and allied services', the Report offered an integrated concept of health centres and domiciliary services in which the traditionally separate hospitals would be but one component.

The Report advocated two types of health centre – primary and secondary. The latter were basically hospitals, staffed by consultants, to be integrated with primary health centres. The former were to house and coordinate all those services in direct contact with the community, such as the doctor, dentist and health visitor. From this primary level 'difficult' cases would be referred upwards to the secondary sector.

The proposed primary health centres would integrate all hitherto separately based domiciliary services, both general practice and municipal. Thus venereal disease clinics and tuberculosis dispensaries would come under the same roof and be staffed by the same personnel as traditional general practice services. The Report consistently stressed the preventive role of the GP: 'to advise how to prevent disease and to improve the conditions of life amongst his patients should be an important element in his work'. The GP would play a valuable part in 'communal services', ante-natal supervision, child welfare, tuberculosis, venereal disease and industrial hygiene. He would be 'mainly domiciliary but partly institutional, mainly individual but partly communal'.[2]

In total, the Dawson Report advocated an integrated structure for the formerly disparate elements of health care. From the domiciliary services in the patient's home to the specialised techniques of the teaching hospital, the Dawson Report proposed a health care structure which would effectively embrace the whole population within its efficient care machinery.

Comprehensive health care

How was it that in a world dominated by independent hospitals the Minister of Health could charge the Dawson Committee with devising a 'systematised' health care provision? How was it possible to envisage 'comprehensive' health care?

The Dispensary vision, in focusing on the space between bodies, made possible both the new socio–medical problems – venereal disease, tuberculosis, child health, the neuroses, etc., and the special clinics which were established to survey the social contacts and often transient geographical manifestations of these mobile pathologies. In this sense the Dawson Report, in advocating an integrated and comprehensive service, constituted a further element in an extended disciplinary apparatus. In as much as the new social diseases and the new manifestations of mental instability were recognised as occurring everywhere, it was obviously desirable to deploy new and extensive forms of health care organisation to cope with these universal epidemics and social threats. A newly constituted social space required a comprehensive medico–social surveillance.

The Dawson Report also represented, at a more general level, the unification of separate fields of visibility. Each of the various components of health care – the new clinics, domiciliary services, general practices and hospitals – which Dawson enveloped in his proposal for a comprehensive system, tended to be limited in their powers of surveillance. For example, the hospital examined the particular bodies in its charge, the school clinic monitored the children for which it had responsibility and the tuberculosis clinics could only keep a watchful eye on those in contact with actual cases of tuberculosis. Within each of these separate medical systems, only certain patients, or only certain parts of patients, were made visible to the observing medical authorities; each system tended to possess its own hierarchies of observation, each its own system of documenting individual cases.

Yet if a line were drawn to link these separate fields of visibility, to integrate their separate hierarchies and coordinate their records, then each single patient and his social space could become more visible, more legible to the medical gaze. The Dawson Report was therefore a proposal for the creation of an integrated and open field of medical visibility. The Report recommended a uniform system of records, throughout the health care system, based on the card index method. A copy of the record would accompany the patient wherever he moved and specially appointed officers would maintain the efficiency of the system: 'such organisation, properly directed, would be of great value in the promotion of national health'.[3]

The National Health Insurance Scheme, of 1911, had instituted a system of record-keeping for all those patients who had a 'panel' doctor, but, because this record was returned to the relevant authorities every year, it was totally inadequate for following through many illnesses. Indeed, such was the poor, if not non-existent, state of patients records, especially in general practice, that quite independently of Dawson a Committee had been appointed by the Ministry of Health to review the whole problem of medical records. In 1920 it too recommended a new system of record-keeping which would enable a continuous record of attendance, diagnosis and treatment to be kept.[4]

A further manifestation of a more open field of visibility is found in the emphasis the Dawson Report placed on physical culture. Indeed, one of the central recommendations of the Dawson Report was for the integration of physical cultures into the health services. Exercise, it was argued, could produce 'a healthy and strong body, with balance and grace of movement; brain control – quick and perfected response and concentration of purpose; the joy of achievement; discipline, playing for the side rather than self, loyalty, comradeship'.[5]

The linking of physical culture with health may be seen to represent the conjoining of two influences. The first is that of space. An emphasis on the space between bodies can be identified in the formal group exercises and in their outdoor setting which became such a familiar sight in the schools, parks and open spaces of Europe in the inter-war years. The distinct and coordinated gestures of arms, legs and bodies reduced the physical mapping of space to the ritualised movement. At the same time, physical culture enabled bodies to be observed. Instead of bodies being confined in homes and hidden by clothing, physical culture enabled them to be legitimately and publicly viewed. To improve the power of this observing eye, the Dawson Report recommended games 'which are free or have an educative design' as well as more formal routine exercises. 'It has been found that the objects aimed at by a formal exercise can often be attained by providing the setting of the game, and with the latter there is a spontaneity and exhilaration absent from the former.'[6]

Exercise was at one and the same time a means of disciplining bodies and a means of expressing that discipline. Exercise in the form of 'drill' had been a panoptic device which had been used to good effect in the army to transform the raw recruit into the disciplined soldier. Similar techniques were employed in the new schools of the late nineteenth century to cope with an analogous problem, the disciplining of unruly children. Exercise had been commended in the Board of Education's 'Suggestions for consideration of teachers' in 1905, but, following a national outcry against purely mechanical drill,[7] a new technique of 'physical training' which recognised the subtleties of disciplining impressionable yet varied bodies was formally advised in the 'Syllabus of physical training for schools' of 1909 and 1919.[8] Physical training, the syllabus pointed out, was entirely different from 'school drill' but it was not total freedom: 'undirected, indiscriminate exercise cannot take the place of a scientific system of physical training';[9] such training, it was felt, would have a physical effect in improving general nutrition, in development of nerve centres in the brain and in correcting poor posture and physical inadequacies, but also an educational effect in developing higher mental and moral qualities.[10]

In short, the 'drill' which had emerged with the Panopticon as a means of analysing individual bodies was replaced by a free yet controlled movement which analysed the relationship between bodies. The Dawson Report, in incorporating this controlled movement of bodies into the new programme of health, further extended the range and power of the medical gaze: 'physical culture is thus concerned with education, with the maintenance of health and the recreation of the people, and with the curing of disease and disability, and there is no sharp line of demarcation between these functions'.[11] An alliance was formally established between the movement of bodies and a regime of hygiene which in the inter-war years gave rise to such varied 'leisure' activities as PT, walking, camping, hiking and nudism and, in the post-war world, to the many bodily exercises undertaken in the name of positive health.

The Pioneer health centre

The Dawson Report had suggested an important role for the GP in preventive medicine. Newman, the Chief Medical Officer at the Ministry of Health, had also felt that while 'all doctors, nurses, midwives, health visitors, sanitary inspectors and welfare workers should be missionaries of hygiene',[12] the GP, especially, was 'the instrument, the outpost, the interpreter', of the new way of health.[13] This perspective was actively supported by Brackenbury, the Secretary of the British Medical Association, who between the wars campaigned vigorously for prevention rather than diagnosis and treatment – the social rather than the clinical (or organic) side of general practice.[14]

Brackenbury gradually shifted BMA policy from supporting a GP role which involved 'curing' in hospital, to caring outside. He argued that the distinguishing feature of a GP case should be home circumstance rather than the severity of the illness. He proposed intermediate 'home hospitals' which would enable the GP to be 'transformed from part-time specialists into part-time social workers'. The GP with his potential intimate knowledge of the patient's family and environment, was ideally placed to monitor the sanitised space of the social. It was to be several decades before Brackenbury's dream practice became realisable but, in the inter-war years, at the point of intersection of this vision of a preventive/social role for the GP, with the open field of visibility as propounded by the Dawson Report, emerged a unique experiment in health care, namely, the Pioneer health centre at Peckham.[15]

An experimental health centre was first opened in 1926 at Peckham at which local families were enrolled and given periodic 'health overhauls'. This screening uncovered much poor health which proved resistant to treatment. The health overhaul, it was concluded, was therefore ineffective 'in the absence of "instruments of health" providing conditions in and through which the biological potentiality of the family can find expression'.[16] The first health centre was therefore closed, funds raised, and a second-stage centre opened in 1935: 'a social structure to be built with a new unit – not the individual but the family'.[17]

In mapping the space created by the interactions of the family, the Peckham health centre offered a conception of health and illness which was primarily social. It advocated 'positive' health as against more traditional 'negative' disease definitions: 'health demands a health consciousness and a health equipment which are distinct and entirely different from the consciousness of disease and the equipment for dealing with either the cure or the prevention of disease'.[18] The seeds of disease, it was believed, were sown in 'disfunction' [*sic*] and disability and these two major disturbances were caused by events in the field of social health.[19] The centre provided no treatment, it was a 'health service of a purely advisory order'.[20]

An ideology of health promotion required new medical techniques and these were provided in screening and surveillance. Families had to undergo three screening procedures on joining the centre. A laboratory and physical examination was followed by a 'family consultation' in which the family was interviewed as a whole unit. The family consultation was found to be especially useful for families on the threshold of change, such as marriage or an impending childbirth.[21] Community surveillance was effected by a novel arrangement. Unlike the other manifestations of the Dispensary in the early twentieth century the Pioneer health centre did not radiate out into the community; instead, it brought the community within its own walls. The social club, which formed such a vital role in the life of the centre, with its attendant games, sports and social activities, acted as both incentive for patients to join the centre and also as a means of surveillance, not the examination of the formal consultation, but the unnoticed silent observation of patients' spontaneous social activity.[22]

These two facets of the Dispensary – disease perceived as a social phenomenon and community surveillance – were, of course, two sides of the same coin. Surveillance discovered disease in the community and this discovery necessitated further surveillance. In effect, the Pioneer health centre destroyed the old distinction between those who were healthy and those who were diseased. Whereas for traditional hospital medicine, illness was a deviant status, to the Dispensary, as found at Peckham, it was normal. If everyone had pathology then everyone would need observing. Thus of everyone attending the health centre only 7% were found to be truly healthy.[23]

The idea that everyone was ill was an important element in the operation of a generalised surveillance. The new social diseases of the twentieth century, tuberculosis, venereal disease and problems of childhood, had been reconstrued to focus medical attention on 'normal' people who were nevertheless 'at risk'. This same notion can also be seen in the discovery of the neuroses which, at least in mild form, came to appear in almost everyone. The innovations of the Peckham centre effectively extended this principle to more traditional organic diseases by dissolving the clear boundary between the healthy and the diseased. This process was to be continued after World War II with the discovery, on the one hand of the 'clinical iceberg' by epidemiologists[24] and, on the other hand of 'illness behaviour' by medical sociologists.[25]

From the institution of a social club to the design of its buildings, every development within the Peckham centre was a conscious attempt to make visible the web of human relations. Every change, every improvement was made with the deliberate aim of extending the observing eye. In 1936, for example, a nursery was added to the facilities: it enabled 'the doctor to make continuous observations on the child in the normal environment'.[26] A special key for use by patients was also designed (though never installed). The key would give access to the building for each individual of every member-family and it would also enable them to gain access to particular facilities within the building. The key, however, was to function in two ways: on the one hand, it would give freedom of access and movement to the patients; on the other, it would enable a record to be kept of these precise comings and goings: 'suppose the scientist should wish to know what individuals are using the swimming bath or consuming milk, the records made by the use of the key give him this information'. The key would at once be important 'for dis-embarrassing the observer of duties connected with control' and 'desirable for freeing the individual member'.[27] Greater freedom could only be met by more invisible and pervasive observation. 'The general visibility and continuity of flow throughout the building is a necessity for the scientist.'[28]

The Peckham experiment was a laboratory for the development, refinement and deployment of new technologies of observation. At

Peckham, individual bodies and their relationships yielded to a clearer field of visibility. 'In the biological laboratories of botany and zoology the microscope has been the main and requisite equipment. The human biologist also requires special "sight" for his field of observation – the family. His new "lens" is the transparency of all boundaries within his field of experiment.'[29]

Social medicine

Following a distinguished career as a consultant physician at Guy's Hospital, John Ryle reached the pinnacle of medical success when he was appointed to the Regius Chair of Physic at Cambridge. In 1943 he resigned this position to become the first Professor of Social Medicine at the newly established Institute of Social Medicine at Oxford.

Social medicine was a new discipline. There had been other forms of social medicine and hygiene but these, as Ryle pointed out, had restricted themselves to various 'deviant' groups, whereas the new social medicine was not so confined.[30] The new social medicine was concerned with the study of people in groups; in particular it searched for social pathology. It embraced 'on the one hand the whole of the activities of public health, administration and of the remedial and allied social services, and on the other the special disciplines necessary for the advancement of knowledge relating to sickness and health in the community'.[31] Hence its important component disciplines were social pathology and hygiology ('the study of health and its causes').[32]

Ryle pointed out that he had spent some 30 years in clinical medicine and during that time disease had been more and more elaborately investigated by mechanical means, to the exclusion of the social domain. The new age had to redress the balance: a new concern with prevention, social pathology and health in the round. 'I submit that we can only do this effectively by electing to pursue the study of social man in sickness and in health.'[33] The new social medicine created an alliance between the old discipline of public health and the new manifestations of the Dispensary, thereby extending the interests of public health from concern with the environment to a concern with social relations.

In its recommendations of 1936 the General Medical Council stated that the medical student should be directed throughout his course to the importance of the measures by which 'normal health' could be assessed and maintained and to the principles and practice of the prevention of disease. In the late 1930s the term 'social medicine', which had previously been used as a general name for municipal health services, came to describe the new discipline which incorporated preventive medicine, public health and a focus on social relationships. Such was the interest that this new subject quickly engendered that the Royal College of Physicians appointed a Social and Preventive Medicine Committee in 1942 'to consider the subject and make recommendations for its development'. An interim report appeared in 1943.[34]

The report pointed out that preventive medicine under the rubric of public health or hygiene was already in the undergraduate medical curriculum, whereas social medicine, in examining the social environment and heredity as they affected health and well-being, represented 'a relatively novel point of view'.[35] The Committee thought that social medicine constituted the background for both preventive and curative medicine and that it was important enough to justify completely reorganising the curriculum to give it its due place. The potential range of social medicine was so broad, however, that much of it would have to be taught – and quite appropriately – in other departments. The obstetrician should teach the preventive as well as the clinical aspect of his subject, as would the paediatrician, the venereologist, the specialist in tuberculosis and the psychiatrist.[36]

An important place in the teaching of social medicine was suggested for the hospital almoner. From an inter-war role of assessing patients' financial means and their ability to contribute towards the cost of treatment, the almoner became caught up in the new task of social investigation and was gradually transposed into the familiar role of the social worker.[37] As a figure, therefore, who emerged from the social domain to police the social, the new hospital almoner was ideally suited to teach social medicine to medical students.

These various suggestions were echoed by the Inter-Departmental Committee on Medical Schools, chaired by Sir William Goodenough, which was appointed by the Minister of Health in 1942 to make recommendations on medical education. A Report was published in 1944 which endorsed most of the recommendations of the Royal College of Physicians' Committee.[38] The Goodenough Report also recognised that social medicine was not restricted to preventive medicine: 'It signifies a particular conception of Medicine; a conception that regards the promotion of health as a primary duty of the doctor, that pays heed to man's social environment and heredity as they affect health, and that recognises that personal problems of health and sickness may have communal as well as individual aspects.' Such a view was receiving increasing support, it was argued, from the medical profession and the general public. 'There is growing support for the view that a general medical practitioner should become the health advisor of his patients and their families and should participate to a greater extent in the conduct of the health services of the country.'[39]

The ideas of social medicine, it was suggested, should 'permeate the whole of medical education'. This would necessitate a fundamental reorientation of that education and of the outlook and methods of most teachers. Anatomy and physiology should not be taught solely such that, by contrast, the pathological could be understood; the study of the normal was important in its own right in the promotion and maintenance of mental and physical health. In the clinical years it was insufficiently recognised that 'in the study of the patient's life as a whole may often be found the reason for his illness and the only key to the restoration of his health. If students are to acquire the right outlook they must see their teachers enlisting the help of almoners, psychiatric social workers, health visitors and other welfare workers, and considering clinical problems against the background of the patient's domestic circumstances and environment.'[40]

The existence of such a social medicine and its various characteristics – concern with the normal and positive health, with screening and social relationships – was a manifestation of an analysable social space between bodies. It was, therefore, at the same moment as a medicine of the social was born that a politics of the social became a possibility. European society throughout the inter-war years was a 'mass' society on which the politics of socialism played in all its varied forms.

If, at the beginning of the nineteenth century when the various elements of the discrete and autonomous body were being fabricated by the panoptic gaze, the ideal project and terrifying dream was signified by Frankenstein's monster, then in the inter-war years it is perhaps Orwell's *1984* or Huxley's *Brave new world* which best express the new configuration of power. The discipline-mechanism, as Foucault clearly states, is 'a functional mechanism that must improve the exercise of power by making it lighter, more rapid, more effective, a design of subtle coercion for a society to come'.[41] Yet how could Orwell's and Huxley's futuristic utopias, which demanded a constant surveillance, a calculated control and the final eclipse of the individual body by the all-pervasive social, be realised either politically or technically?

The solution to this problem emerged during the war at a point when it became politically possible to create an exhaustive surveillance machinery. In the armed forces, where fighting efficiency had to be sustained, an experimental ground was created for the emergence of new techniques of observation. As Crewe, Professor of Public Health and Social Medicine in Edinburgh and a brigadier in the army medical service acknowledged, 'the Army with its all-in system of medical inspection and care has provided unique opportunities for the rapid development of social medicine'.[42] In the army, health promotion and disease prevention had to be coordinated with and seen in the context of other functions such as planning, organisation, welfare, training, etc. Thus, from the outset, social medicine in the army 'demanded for its development a corpus of knowledge concerning occupation, locality, social amenities, personal habits, aspirations, risks and responsibilities': in short, a science of human ecology.[43]

On the domestic front, the war gave 'a new impetus to all forms of health education' as the Chief Medical Officer to the Ministry of Health reported.[44] Increased publicity was given to health and it could be claimed that 'more than ever before, health, in contradistinction to disease, is news, and prevention is acquiring some of the drama of cure'.[45] Yet, while a medicine of the social was promoted by a war-time need to know and make visible the social networks of the community under threat, it was also the product of another movement which acted to reinforce the Dispensary system of community surveillance and make its workings far more efficient. That new development was to be found in the invention of the survey.

5

Technologies of the survey

In 1839 the Poor Law Commissioners were given the task of surveying the sanitary conditions of the 'labouring classes'. Data were gathered from boards of guardians, medical officers of unions and general practitioners and published in 1842 as a *Report on the sanitary conditions of the labouring population of Great Britain.* In 1851 the Census in England and Wales made an attempt to count the number of blind and deaf and dumb in the community and the number of lunatics in asylums. Both these surveys represented attempts to gain knowledge of aspects of the population but both were limited. The Poor Law Commissioners' survey relied mainly on qualitative data, as did later surveys such as that of the Health of Towns Commission of 1844. The Census, on the other hand, obtained quantitative data but under-reporting was recognised as a serious problem, especially after 1871 when questions on whether imbeciles, idiots or lunatics lived in the household were introduced.

Further refinements in survey technique were made in Booth's *Life and labour of the people of London: 1892–1903*, in which information, including data on sickness, was obtained through the agency of the London School Board visitors on every family in 3400 London streets. Rowntree's survey of poverty in York, which commenced in 1899 dispensed with intermediaries and gathered data directly from respondents. A survey of poverty by Bowley in five provincial towns in 1912 introduced sampling by selecting one in twenty households, at equal intervals, from a complete list. Thus, by the second decade of the twentieth century, sufficient techniques had been developed to make the survey an efficient instrument for the investigation and measurement of populations.[1]

The Dispensary had emerged in the same years as survey methodology was refined, early in the twentieth century. The Dispensary mapped both geographical and social space and therefore functioned as an apparatus of surveillance. In its ceaseless monitoring of the community, it represented, in somewhat rudimentary form, a survey. The possibility therefore arose of fusing the particular techniques of surveillance that had been developed in survey methodology with a system of disciplinary power that was embodied in the Dispensary. The survey, a mechanism for 'measuring' reality, could be transformed into a technology for the 'creation' of reality; the tactics of the survey could make the operation of disciplinary power throughout a society more effective and more efficient.

Foucault points out that a menagerie had been constructed at Versailles in which a central room, the king's salon, looked out onto seven cages containing different species of animals so that the king, from a single vantage point, might oversee his animal collection.[2] It would thus seem that the particular architectural structure that Bentham succeeded in marrying to a system of power was already in existence before the invention of the Panopticon. Similarly, during the early decades of the twentieth century, a mechanism for the investigation of communities, in the form of the survey, existed side by side with a device (the Dispensary) which enabled the gaze to be deployed throughout the community, without the one assimilating the other. Indeed, when survey techniques were finally harnessed to the Dispensary, it was not because it was realised that the survey might improve the efficiency, range and invisibility of the mechanisms of power as embodied in the Dispensary; that discovery was to come later. The interest of the Dispensary in survey techniques arose in the inter-war years from its central concern with the normal.

The normal control

The idea of the norm was, as Foucault argues, a particular invention of the Panopticon.[3] The examination of bodies involved the approximation and comparison of each body with the 'normal' since the Panopticon was concerned to identify deviants who failed to measure up to the norm. The distinction between those who met the norm and those who did not was, however, absent from the Dispensary. Instead of being an arbitrary external referrent, the normal came to be located within the social body itself: bodies themselves defined normality. A central element in the functioning of the Dispensary came to be the rejection of 'the norm' and the focus on 'normal variability'.

In 1930, Thomas Lewis had commended to his colleagues the value of 'clinical science'.[4] He argued that medicine, through the exaggerated importance it attached to diagnosis, had come to over-depend on techniques of clinical observation. In the part these techniques had been valuable and had led to major advances, but, as Lewis observed, 'eventually the fertility of this method greatly declines by a process of exhaustion, and, for those who can read the signs, this time has come in medicine'.[5] In place of the observational method, Lewis proposed clinical science which would use the experimental method.

The clinical science campaign, which, from 1930 onwards,was actively promoted by Lewis, placed the body of the patient in a new context. Lewis challenged the norms by which the body had been defined. Curative medicine, he argued, dealt with the individual while clinical science, or 'progressive medicine', was collective in its outlook. To the latter the patient was 'but an incident ... one who exhibits phenomena of disease to be compared and correlated with those displayed by other subjects'.[6] In effect, the normalising judgement of the clinical gaze, in this new progressive medicine, would not use 'the norm' as a referrent but instead place the body of the patient in the context of 'other subjects' and then measure the differences.

The comparison, moreover, was not only with other patients, but also with the healthy. In the past, the pathological or the abnormal had stood in opposition to the physiological or normal. In clinical science, however, applied physiology was used to explain the pathological: in other words, explanation by reference to the normal came to invest the explanation of the abnormal. The possibility of a relational medicine was explored as the body of the patient was analysed in juxtaposition to other bodies, both healthy and sick.

At the same time as the body of the patient was placed in its new social context, it also, through the identification of particular differences, became further individuated. Lewis, for example, argued that in certain situations the patient need not be compared with the healthy but with himself: 'You may study heart failure by comparing normal subjects with those who show failure. It is not the same thing; it is the chance of minutely comparing the normal and the abnormal states of circulation *in one and the same subject* that is so important: here is the perfect control.'[7]

Use of the patient as his own control – which furthered the constitution of a relational medicine – can also be seen in the emphasis given to the physiological basis of symptoms. Symptoms, from being the subjective and therefore unreliable component of the diagnostic process (signs being objective), were examined in the context of physiological processes: 'the study of symptoms necessitates very close consideration of the relevant mechanisms of the body while this is working naturally'.[8] The patient, instead of simply describing the occurrence of symptoms, was asked to come under observation while the symptom was 'provoked' and changes in body functioning monitored and observed.

This close examination of the apparently pathological, in the terms of the physiological, produced anomalies. Ryle, for example, in investigating the physiologically normal of the population, had discovered that 10% of fit medical students showed gastric acidity which would previously have been regarded as abnormal.[9] As Ryle was later to point out, this led him to believe that 'a similar variability may be demonstrated or assumed in respect of all measurable physiological activities and of other immeasurable physical, mental, and emotional states and processes'.[10]

These problems in the variability of normal and disease states were particularly pertinent to therapeutics. The success of many established therapies was based on the '*post hoc ergo propter hoc*' fallacy whereby the natural course of the disease was mistakenly attributed to the treatment. But what was the natural or normal course of a disease? Clinical science could in part answer the question by observing the common features in the natural histories of various diseases but this rarely had predictive value in therapeutics.

In the 1930s the '*post hoc propter hoc*' fallacy was placed in a new context: not simply as the adage of the sceptical clinician but as a part of a strategy which sought to examine the natural or normal course of disease. Hence there emerged the two great twentieth-century inventions of therapeutics, the placebo and the control. The concept of the placebo emerged in medical discourse in the context of the apparent efficacy of pharmacologically inert substances; the 'normal' control became the referrent for pharmacological activity in the body of the patient.

Shapiro has traced the first use of the word placebo, in its current medical sense, to the beginning of the nineteenth century.[11] However, the term was used so infrequently that Wood's *Therapeutics*, whose fourteen editions covered the period from 1875 to 1908, never indexed it.[12] Indeed, Shapiro has been able to discover only one medical paper between 1900 and 1930 which actually used the word and that paper was primarily about ethics. Between 1930 and 1950 there were seven papers about the placebo effect and between 1950 and 1957 some 48 papers which in some way discussed it.

This growing interest in the placebo effect can be seen to have arisen at the point of intersection of several influences. Firstly, the placebo, unlike the active drug, did not in principle interfere with the natural or normal course of the disease: it was therefore of value to a clinical gaze which sought to examine the normal. Secondly, the placebo effect was seen as having great power itself because it unlocked the power of individuals over their own bodies – this latter being the essence of the disciplinary power of panoptic and Dispensary visions. Thirdly, an interest in the placebo led both to the importance of having 'normal' controls in therapeutic trials and to the use of placebos within those trials. The history of the controlled clinical trial, as well as being a record of therapeutic improvement, can also be read as the refinement and development of an analysis of the normal patient in the context of a disciplinary apparatus.

In 1931, the Medical Research Council created the Therapeutics Trial Committee to test under 'controlled conditions' the efficacy of new drugs developed by companies in the British Association of Chemical Manufacturers. During the 1930s, various therapies were tested under the auspices of the MRC and by 1943 the *Lancet* could write: 'Our experience of the last few years proves that writers on clinical subjects are more figure conscious than their elder brothers. It is less common to find startling conclusions from (say) six cases.'[13] A year later, after a well-controlled trial of patulin in the common cold had shown no significant difference between control and experimental groups, the *Lancet* concluded that the lesson of the enquiry was that 'no remedy for colds must be judged until it has been submitted to a large scale trial'.[14]

The study, often judged the most important of these early researches, was that of the MRC trial of streptomycin in tuberculosis.[15] The first trial of streptomycin in tuberculous meningitis did not use controls as the infection was invariably lethal.[16] However, in the second part of the trial, to test the effectiveness of streptomycin in pulmonary tuberculosis, untreated controls were added as the course of the disease was unpredictable.[17]

The *British Medical Journal* devoted a leader to this 'controlled therapeutic trial' an idea, it thought, 'recent enough to call new'. In describing the design of the investigation, the *Journal* was at pains to reaffirm the integrity of the radiologists who had read the x-rays not knowing from which group the patient had come: 'it in no way questions the intellectual honesty of the investigator who is thus asked to work "blind"'.[18] The *Lancet* thought the study was brought 'as near to a laboratory experiment as is practicable and makes it unique in the dismal history of tuberculosis chemotherapeutic trials'.[19]

The invention of the controlled clinical trial, in which the normal population became the referrent for monitoring the course of disease in individuals,[20] also necessitated the development of appropriate statistics for comparing experimental and control groups. In 1937 the *Lancet* had invited Bradford Hill to prepare a series of articles on basic medical statistics, as it was felt that the medical profession was insufficiently conscious of the need to express its findings in number and was often unaware of the importance of taking into consideration unknown and uncontrollable variables.[21] Following its success, the series was published as a book later that same year.[22]

The development of statistical methods and the concept of the normal control population also released epidemiology from its 'experimental' cul-de-sac. Earlier in the century, Greenwood & Topley had revived a quiescent epidemiology with an experimental approach.[23] The focus of these early twentieth-century epidemiologists was not so much the infective danger of the environment but, like that of so many disciples of the Dispensary, the health dangers of social contact. Experimental epidemiology was, therefore, concerned with 'crowd diseases' and the study of the transmission of diseases throughout populations.[24] Rats and mice were used to simulate the vagaries of human relationships, over-crowding, distances, proximities, etc., and precise mathematical summaries were devised, especially of the 'epidemic wave', to express the path of infections as they were passed from animal to animal through the colony.[25]

The invention of the human control population enabled epidemiology to focus once more on human populations and the 'experiment' to be reproduced in patients. The case-control study, in which the sick are compared (usually retrospectively) with control cases, was used by Lane-Clayton in the 1920s to study the outcome of treatment of breast cancer.[26] But perhaps its best-known early use was in Doll & Hill's work, published in 1950, linking lung cancer and cigarette smoking.[27]

The effect of the normal control was to place the patient and his disease, treatment and prognosis, in a social and conceptual space which encompassed the social body. There was not a hospital wall between the ill and the community but a measurable and calculable gap and it was, increasingly, only by placing the patient in a field invested by the normal (derived from the social body) that the patient could be either known or constituted. The corollary was that the social body itself had to be further made visible and subject to the clinical gaze.

Knowledge of populations was promoted by further refinements in recording techniques in the inter-war years. The Medical Research Council, for example, had devised special charts for its inter-war School Epidemic Investigation which enabled the movement of disease within a population to be recorded, and Pickles, the Wensleydale GP, used a modified version of these same charts for his now classic observations on the course, natural history and distribution of various diseases in the 1930s.[28]

Mechanical tabulation of hospital records was developed and in 1936 Spear & Gould suggested it now provided a 'powerful agent in the hands of the investigator. In this direction we feel that the almost limitless possibilities of the system have not been and are not realised.' These techniques, they felt, would also be applicable to surveys of disease in populations.[29]

The Nuffield Trust had funded a Bureau of Health and Sickness Records to undertake morbidity studies in the Oxford region. The Bureau devoted considerable energy to 'developing and standardising better recording systems for use in research departments, hospitals and the public health service'.[30] In 1943, under the new Institute of Social Medicine at Oxford, it attempted to measure total morbidity in the population, using both hospital and GP records.

A classification of morbidity was also developed through the Nuffield

Provincial Hospitals Trust and the Editorial Board for the Official Medical History of the War. A special MRC Committee was appointed which checked the in-patient records of the emergency medical service hospitals and from them developed a classification system which enabled morbidity data on all military personnel entering the EMS hospitals to be coded and card indexed.[31]

The focus of these improvements in coding and recording techniques was twofold: on the one hand, they offered a chance to assess the natural course of disease in the population, unencumbered by medical intervention, and, on the other hand, then enabled the normal to be more fully investigated. Ryle summed up the central problems with the title of his essay 'The meaning of normal and the measurement of health'.[32]

Whereas disease could be observed in separate individuals, health was a concept that could only be constructed from populations. Yet such was the range of normal, as Ryle pointed out, that 'only in living samples of sufficient size can we usefully observe in juxtaposition and compare the manifestations of health and sickness and borderline states'. The source of these living samples could not be the hospital ward but must be the 'welfare centres and nurseries, in schools and universities, in the armed forces, or the large communities'.[33]

The focus on the wider community, which characterised the Dispensary, was considerably enhanced by the war. The war presented a community under threat; a community which had to be united behind the war effort and at the same time monitored for potential weaknesses; a community which had to be analysed to see whether its strengths and resources were being adequately used. In short, the perception of the problems of war-time created problems of social threat similar to those faced earlier in the century by the reformers in the midst of epidemics of tuberculosis and venereal diseases. Here was a problem which demanded an improved rigour in the disciplinary mechanisms of the society: this need was met by the deployment of a new technology, namely, the medico–social survey.

Surveillance by the survey

It would be inaccurate to argue that the medico–social survey was invented during the war. Such surveys had been conducted during the nineteenth century, though the development of adequate quantitative methodology had not occurred until early in the twentieth century. Thereafter, occasional surveys had been conducted. Some of the earlier studies were repeated: Bowley repeated his 'Five town survey', of 1912, in 1923–4; the London School of Economics conducted a survey in 1928 – some three decades after Booth's pioneering work – entitled *New survey of London life and labour*, and the University of Liverpool, in 1929, produced the *Merseyside survey* which included aspects of illness in the community.[34]

The newly created Ministry of Health had resolved, in 1920, to use survey techniques in the elucidation of problems of public health in the same way as had nineteenth-century investigators. 'We must pursue this method . . . but we must make our surveys more comprehensive.'[35] A study on the incidence of rheumatic diseases based on data collected from a group of insurance medical practitioners was published in 1924.[36] Surveys of the adequacy of public health services in different countries were inaugurated following the Local Government Act of 1929.[37] In 1933, researches were commenced into the nature of the diet in different parts of the country, the results of studying the diets of 69 working class families in Newcastle being published in 1936.[38] The effect of the 'normal' diet was also analysed by haemoglobin level surveys. Haemoglobin levels were measured in school children in Manchester, Warrington, Barnsley and Huddersfield and levels in pre-school children and their mothers were established in Warrington, Barnsley and Leeds.[39]

Other attempts to survey the community – though often without formal survey techniques – were also made in the inter-war period. The Pioneer health centre at Peckham had attempted to map the health of its population during the 1930s by careful recording, monitoring and surveillance.[40] Madge & Harrisson had founded Mass Observation in 1937 with the express purpose of providing a voice for the ordinary member of the community. Amateur 'observers' were appointed around the country 'to describe fully, clearly and in simple language all that he sees and hears in connection with the specific problem he is asked to work on'.[41] These various surveys and quasi-surveys, however, supplied only limited and unclear pictures: it was the advent of the war that created the conditions for a greater visibility and a concomitant, more penetrating and unified gaze, over the whole community.

The war-time community presented various social problems, among them dislocation of labour, war injuries, evacuation, nutrition and rationing. If the war was to be won, a firm grasp had to be taken over the nation's functioning. And if medicine was to play its part in this great effort then it would have to provide medical services for the whole population and know more about the distribution and extent of medical need. As Langdon-Brown argued: 'What is needed is a complete sequence of medical supervision throughout life.'[42]

In 1940 the Ministry of Information, through the National Institute of Economic and Social Research, created a 'public opinion testing machine' called the War-time Social Survey.[43] The *Lancet* pointed out that such 'new methods of studying the population would be helpful, not only in planning legislation but also in watching the effects of totalitarian war on the community as a whole'.[44] The War-time Social Survey offered 'direct access to the raw material of government, the people themselves'.[45] Random samples of the population were interviewed for their knowledge and attitudes towards various subjects. Members of the public were found 'willing, and even enthusiastic' to provide information.[46] The government could, therefore, at one and the same time know the effect of food publicity, the attitude to news broadcasts, the fact that 67% of the population believed the purpose of the war was to protect liberty and freedom, 6% to save civilisation and that 2% expressed 'cynical views'.[47]

Knowledge of public opinion could then be integrated with other surveys of the population. A network of surveillance, for example, began to be constructed to make visible the nutritional state of the community. The Chief Medical Officer at the Ministry of Health later contended: 'In order to be able to advise on matters of nutritional policy it was necessary for the Ministry of Health to keep a continuous watch on the nutritional state of the people.'[48] In 1940 the Ministry of Health revived the dietary surveys of the 1930s on a regular basis; a clinical survey of malnutrition was conducted in 1942; the Medical Research Council commenced community surveys of blood haemoglobin; a survey of the height and weight of 12 000 children was carried out in 1940; a controlled trial of the nutritional value of supplementary vitamins was carried out in 1940 on 2500 school children.[49]

In the past, government departments had collected some statistics by means of a return. These 'returns' were limited in scope, slow to collect and remained uncoordinated between different departments. The survey drew together these incidental statistics into a coherent map. Departments could supplement their statistical returns and relate one set of data to another by sample surveys. 'There is no doubt that in this way a most flexible instrument for the compilation of a wide range of statistics can be developed.'[50]

It became possible to coordinate hospital data. Between 1940 and 1946 every fifth patient in the emergency medical service was coded. The Medical Research Council provided a Provisional Classification of Diseases and Injuries, in 1943, to enable appropriate codings of morbidity[51] and in 1949 this procedure was formalised in the Hospital In-patient Morbidity Survey.

But what of the general health of the community? There had been reports of a great increase in minor morbidity and of over-crowded general practitioner surgeries.[52] In 1944 the Social Survey was extended to encompass the perceived health of the population. A random sample of the civilian population was regularly interviewed at two-monthly intervals about their health in the preceding three months. The results provided constant information about the extent – and changes – of illness in the population and data on use of medical services.[53] The government was thus able to monitor the health of the population in regularly up-dated health indices and the Chief Medical Officer at the Ministry of Health advocated further studies. There was a need for surveillance of pregnant women: perhaps this could be possible through providing detachable slips in ration books? There was, moreover, a need for a 'statistical framework linking maternity, paediatrics and school medical services to one another and to adult health services'.

The comprehensive surveillance network that the survey deployed throughout the community should not be interpreted as simply a device for social control. Certainly, in as much as it was a disciplinary apparatus it was concerned with ordering a population, but this was only one component of its overall functioning. The survey was also an apparatus of normalisation. It deliberately sought out the normal population and measured it. The survey, as Ryle was to argue, was a means of measuring the health and illness of the 'total person'. Doctors had for too long made judgements based on constant association with sick people and advanced disease; most lacked 'the experience of examining large numbers of ostensibly healthy children, adolescents, or adults'. He therefore proposed the medical examination of large, randomly selected populations, measuring height, weight, haemoglobin, blood pressure, pulse-rate, x-ray, personality, intelligence, skin complexion, fatness, adaptability, etc.[55]

In effect, the survey established the possibility of removing the abnormal/normal divide. The survey classified bodies on a continuum: there were no inherent distinctions between a body at one end and one at the other, their only differences were the spaces which separated them. The referrent external to the population under study – the norm – which had for almost two centuries governed the analysis and distribution of bodies was replaced by the relative positions of all bodies. The survey was a synthesised gaze to relationships, to the gaps between people.

Like the Panopticon, the survey was therefore a two-edged sword. It was an instrument of order and control, a technique for managing the distribution of bodies and preventing their potentially dangerous mixings. On the other hand, this ordering required the identification of relationships through the confession of the body. Illness was no longer the preserve of the medical profession but of the body's own perceptions; the body had to speak, not of some abstract pathological theory of illness, but of immediate feelings. Thus, while the survey became increasingly concerned with the 'objectification' of personal experience through its constant measurement and analysis, it must not be forgotten that those same personal experiences were a fabrication of the creative component of the survey which demanded their visibility. At the very moment as the Survey of Sickness established its intricate net of surveillance over the whole community it was therefore met by a rising crescendo of individual expression.

The survey provided a technological instrument of surveillance which enabled the Dispensary perspective to increase its deployment throughout the community. The survey at once solved the technical problems of examining – and knowing over time – the normal population, and both the ephemeral and chronic health problems arising within it. 'Health, like disease, is never a static process', Ryle argued. 'Alike in the individual and in communities it varies quantitatively from day to day and year to year. If we are to secure its upward trend we must know of its manifestations, its incidence, and its aetiology, and the study of each of these requires the employment of methods of measurement and comparison.'[56] Survey information, it was thought, might be the basis for 'a system whereby the Ministry of Health could promote preventive measures at the outset of an epidemic much more speedily and effectively than is now possible'.[57]

The survey could provide standards for use in clinical work and in individual health assessments. It would enable socio–medical comparisons of privileged and underprivileged groups and of changes over time. 'Surely the health of the people, too, is now worthy of more detailed inquiry. Without more precise knowledge we cannot effectually ensure the proper supervision of health in the home, the school, the workshop, the armed forces, and the nation as a whole.'[58]

The survey made a truly social medicine a realisable goal. Social medicine 'might be much assisted by analysing information about illness in relation to environmental factors, occupation and age, which the survey method makes possible'.[59] At the Institute of Social Medicine at Oxford, Ryle instituted a major survey of child health, observing the health of children registered in the town at birth through to the age of five. Radiographic studies were pursued to show the wide range of normal variability; occupational morbidity and accidents in local factories were monitored; a five-year study of the health of students at two colleges of the University was commenced.[60]

The survey was an instrument of community surveillance through which the bodies of both sick and well could be caught up in a web of observation. The Panopticon had been an invention in the order of power similar in importance to the invention of the steam engine in the order of production.[61] The survey represented a further significant development in the refinement of the gaze, in the generation and maintenance of total visibility. In the survey, a system of power, which was not restricted by the walls of certain institutions but extended throughout the community, was married to various methodological principles to create a new and more efficient technology of power.

Surveys had been carried out in the past without their value to a system of power being appreciated. War provided the conditions for the new alliance to be forged and, in particular, for the virtues of the sample survey to become apparent. The sample survey both depended on, and in some ways forced, recognition of the normal. The homogeneity and heterogeneity of populations was seen to vary and 'the methods of sampling must be adapted to the populations under study'.[62] The sample survey also embodied the panoptic principle of inverted visibility: all seeing yet unseen. 'A measure is made,' noted the *Lancet*, 'while the vast multitude to whom it applies, whether human or cellular, swirls by, unaware that it has been measured.'[63]

The survey therefore constituted an apparatus for distributing the effects of a disciplinary gaze throughout society; a device for individualising through measuring the differences between people; a means of constructing healthy bodies through its analysis of the normal. The survey, like the Panopticon before it, 'atomizes and disindividualizes' power.[64] Power had its principle, not so much in a person, as in a certain distribution of 'bodies, surfaces, lights, gazes'. Hence, it little mattered who constituted the observing authorities for they in their turn were bound up with the workings of this new machine. It is not therefore surprising to discover that all the staff at the Institute of Social Medicine at Oxford were themselves medically examined once a year.[65]

6

Disciplines of the survey: 1. child life and health

In establishing a new political economy of power the Panopticon had created a conceptual domain and an architectural space which required policing. During the early nineteenth century a unified medical profession emerged to take on this role. In similar fashion the extensive deployment of the survey in post-war medicine produced changes and realignments in both the form of medical knowledge and the organisation of the medical profession.

Perhaps, when the history of the sociology of the medical profession comes to be written from post-war sociological texts and journals, the apparent diversity of analytical perspectives – from liberal to repressive – will be seen to be simply different components of an overall system of disciplinary power.[1] Equally, the diversity of views which have characterised the explanation of medical specialisation ('an inevitable and desirable accompaniment of medical advance', through to simply a device for professional advancement[2]) can be embraced in an analysis which examines, not medical knowledge, but its object. It is the gaze which at once unifies medical knowledge and maintains its fragmentations. The various specialties which have emerged, surgical, medical, pathological, investigative, far from being somewhat 'random' events,[3] all relate to aspects of the detailed examination and analysis of the body: in short, the panoptic vision is inscribed into the very structure of medical knowledge and its social organisation. Thus when the survey established new zones of visibility it thereby created the space for the observing gaze of new disciplines.

Surveys of childhood

In 1940 there were two medicines for children. First, there was the direct manifestation of the Dispensary as found in child welfare clinics, milk depots, nursery schools, the school medical service, etc., which monitored the community and spread the new hygiene.[4] The second was the relatively new specialty of paediatrics, a direct outgrowth of clinical medicine.[5]

An interest in diseases of children had been shown by some general physicians from the late nineteenth century.[6] This specialist interest was justified in the main by the apparently peculiar presentation of various diseases in childhood. Forsyth expressed this view in his *Children in health and disease*, of 1909, when he stated: 'With few exceptions the pathological processes of youth and of maturity are alike ... clinical effects however differ.'[7] The name given to the Society for the Study of Diseases in Children, founded in 1901, signified the subsidiary position of the child relative to the disease. Hutchinson, one of the first general physicians to take an interest in diseases of childhood, confessed that had his practice been solely restricted to children his knowledge of children's diseases would have been 'poorer and meaner'.[8]

With the child as an object of increasing concern, and the invention of the 'problem child' in the early twentieth century[9], the medical gaze shifted towards the diseases peculiar to children rather than the unusual manifestation of 'adult diseases' in children. The British Paediatric Association, founded in 1928, was born of this view and by the 1940s it had become the rule rather than the exception for physicians in the diseases of children to confine themselves to that specialty. In effect, a mere side-interest of general physicians became a specialty in its own right through the elaboration of childhood and childhood relationships. Yet the focus on childhood remained essentially a focus on a figure in the Panopticon, in that inter-war paediatrics reproduced the cognitive and organisational forms of its parent medical discipline. Meetings, for example, at the Section for the Study of Diseases in Children, and research reported in *Archives of Disease in Childhood*, were all wholly concerned with the examination of the characteristics of the individual case.[10]

A major realignment in paediatrics began to occur during World War II when the paediatrician's gaze shifted from the child as a figure in the Panopticon to the child in the community: children were evacuated; food for children was in short supply and the threat of malnutrition loomed; children were stressed by disruption of families and loss of parents. The problem was no longer the place of the disease in its nosology but of the child in its community and social context. As Jameson, Chief Medical Officer at the Ministry of Health argued 'in the past paediatrics had shown too little interest in child development and had rather confined their attention to the sick child'.[11] The techniques of the public health child health services ('periodical medical examination coupled with surveillance of a less formal kind'[12]) would now need to be learned and deployed by a community orientated paediatrics.

During the war, paediatricians meeting at the Royal Society of Medicine increasingly discussed the problems of the child in the community.

Discussions were held on the problems of the evacuated child, the role of child guidance, the effects of war-time rationing on child health, nutritional anaemia in children, the decline in breast feeding and the future of the school medical services.[13] The child in the war-time community had to be constantly observed, data recorded and health care organised.

Yet how were these various facets of the social life of childhood to be made known? How could malnutrition be recognised? How could emotional disturbance be identified? There were two problems. One was the problem of the normal child, which was to dominate post-war paediatrics – What were the normal dietary requirements? What was the normal haemoglobin level? What was normal psychological adjustment? The second problem was, given these critieria of normality, how were deviations and variations in children to be picked up? The solution to both problems was the survey.

The new perception of the child, as a figure within the social domain, immediately brought to the attention of paediatricians the lack of data on normal children. In a discussion of the effects of war-time rationing on children at the Royal Society of Medicine, unpublished data from a dietary survey of 1000 middle class children, between 1935 and 1939, were brought to the notice of members.[14] Data from a small group of children of parents in the professions in Newcastle, published by Newcastle Corporation Health Department, were used in a discussion of nutritional anaemia.[15] The shortage of good-quality published data was apparent and, during the war years, the first moves were made to correct this deficiency.

Starting in the autumn of 1941 the haemoglobin levels of a group of normal woman and children were collected so that, by 1942, 550 women and 850 children had been recorded.[16] A study from Birmingham reported that 2698 children had been breast-fed in the first quarter of 1942 compared with 1937 in the first quarter of 1941.[17] A nutritional survey of school children in Oxfordshire, London and Birmingham was undertaken by the Oxford Nutrition Survey of the Institute of Social Medicine in 1943.[18] Gradually, these observations of the social body of the child came to supplement the examination of the individual case and paediatric knowledge became based, not only on clinical phenomena, but also on social facts.

It rapidly became apparent that perhaps the greatest ignorance was of normal growth and development. The height and weight of a child could not be judged by the traditional clinical method of approximation to a nosological category, for, given the apparent range of normal variability, there were no criteria by which that category could be sustained. The only viable referrent would be other children but this would require knowledge of the full range of heights and weights of all normal children.

In 1942 the Executive Committee of the British Paediatric Association established a Sub-Committee to investigate the feasibility of a height and weight survey of the population. There was initially some difficulty in obtaining funding: the Science Committee of the Royal College of Physicians declined to help, as did the Nuffield Foundation. In 1949 a new Committee was established to conduct a survey of growth in children, this time in cooperation with the Ministries of Health and Education.[19]

In the meantime, other studies were carried out. Observations on the growth of children were reported from the Institute of Social Medicine at Oxford.[20] A study of the relation of puberty to height and weight was published.[21] A retrospective study of the relationship of birth weight to mental development was presented to the AGM of the British Paediatric Association in 1948.[22] Yet, as Faulkner pointed out with some impatience in 1952, these various studies were open to criticism and until longitudinal findings were reported 'there was no simple satisfactory test of normal growth in the human child';[23] equally, there was no technique by which the outline of the normal child could be fabricated.

In 1964, looking back over the growth of paediatrics, MacKeith noted that the 'most remarkable single change in paediatric practice in the last 20 years is that today a paediatrician's routine examination nearly always includes some estimate of the child's development'.[24] The major innovations that had enabled the realisation of this procedure were the growth curves and percentile charts derived from the findings of the post-war longitudinal studies.[25] Whereas pre-war paediatrics had viewed the child as a solitary figure in the Panopticon, to be observed, described and analysed, post-war paediatrics, through the technology of the survey, placed the child against the background of the social body – essentially to be compared. The sick body of the child was no longer to be constructed by a clinical gaze which sought to analyse in the context of nosological referrents, but by a gaze over the normal child against whom, by juxtaposition, the sick child was created.

The discovery of the normal child as the context for paediatric judgements posed an immediate problem, however. A test of normal growth assumed the possibility of abnormal growth: yet, how, from knowledge of other childrens' growth, could the boundaries of normality be identified? When was a single point on the growth and weight chart, to which the sick child was reduced, to be construed as abnormal? The questions seemed important yet they could not be answered from the percentile chart. The problem was that the questions themselves belonged to an alternative paradigm, a perceptual gaze which sub-divided the world of childhood into normal and abnormal. An inherent characteristic of the survey – and of the Dispensary – was that it distributed variables continuously within the social domain and, while it was possible to declare one child 'shorter than average' or 'only in the second percentile', it was obviously entirely arbitrary to declare such a finding abnormal.

Thus, in the immediate post-war period, while those paediatricians who functioned in a Dispensary apparatus demanded the technologies and findings of the survey, those who maintained a more limited view of the child's body found the survey confused matters rather than clarified them. Bransby of the Ministry of Health had opposed the British Paediatric Association's proposed war-time survey of height and weight on the grounds that it would serve 'no useful purpose as no conclusions could be drawn from it'.[26] Later, in 1950, he still insisted that the boundaries of abnormality should be imposed on the survey: it is 'not sufficient simply to set statistical limits to normality; a standard must stand up to clinical test'.[27] Yet how could a clinical gaze, which examined the state of the individual child, be consonant with a perception which reduced the child to a point or line on the growth and weight chart? The child as located on the chart, in its social context, necessitated a 'naked-eye judgement' which explicitly accepted that the 'definition of abnormality must be "arbitrary"'.[28] While the survey had seemed to promise the identification and recognition of abnormality in the community, its actual effect had been to confound it. Douglas, reporting on his national longitudinal study started in 1948, pointed out that his findings about the heights and weights of two-year-olds were of no value in isolating 'those who have suffered from ill-health, poor home conditions, or inefficient maternal care', nor was it possible to be predictive from them.[29]

Thus the survey began to weaken the boundary between normality and abnormality in childhood. It seemed to the paediatrician that this posed problems for the identification of the abnormal child; the corollary was that normality became essentially problematic. In effect, the survey which sought to map the social body had identified its own set of problems which further justified its extension. The result was twofold: an increasing reliance on the survey as an instrument of research in paediatrics and a new discourse on the normal child.

Problems of the normal child

In 1953 Illingworth published the first edition of his classic text, *The normal child*.[30] He pointed out that, at that time, it could not be said that knowledge of the normal child was an essential basis for the study of the sick and diseased child, but that he felt there was a need to know considerable variations of normal. By the second edition of 1957 he could note the 'increasing interest in the problems of the normal child'.[31]

The 'problems of the normal child' would have been a contradiction in terms for the Panopticon, but, for the Dispensary, all children were normal in that they belonged to the social body: it was the problems of the social body, as they manifested themselves through the sick child, that informed this new medical perception. The Panopticon had constituted bodies through examining their abnormalities, the Dispensary constituted them through locating them in the community, in their social context, embedded in a network of relationships. Thus, whereas the gaze of the pre-war years had invented particular problems of the child (delicate, nervous, solitary, neuropathic, etc.), the paediatrics of the post-war world, in focusing on relationships of childhood, invented the series of problems which were located in their social environment – the battered child, the deprived child, the neglected child, the abused child. Pre-war, the child was essentially constituted by analysis of discrete bodies and problems were located *within* the child; post-war, the child was increasingly constituted by its social mapping in the community and its problems were located *around* the child. In 1964, for example, Illingworth argued that the idea of the maladjusted child was inappropriate: 'it is the parents who are maladjusted not the child'.[32]

In the post-war world the normal child came to invest the body of the sick child. Disease could not be identified in isolation: the normal child of three was very different from the normal child of ten. 'Manifestations of one and the same disorder may differ in patients of different age. What is abnormal at one period of life may be normal at another. Symptoms, signs, and the results of investigations have to be interpreted in the light of the patient's age and maturity.... In its broad ambit paediatrics must necessarily include such diverse aspects of growth as the biochemical and immunological, the intellectual, emotional and social.'[33]

The normal child, as constituted by the investigation of growth and development, pervaded the diseased child. On the one hand, within the diseased child, 'the natural inherent struggle to maintain or regain growth can be seen to have its influence on the disease process itself'.[34] It remained for the paediatrician 'to decide whether the derangement from the average is of quantitative importance. Why is the boy below average height, and should he be given testosterone? Is the factor in this girl's obesity constitutional, endocrine or emotional, and should a carbohydrate-restricted diet be imposed upon her? Is this child's failure to gain weight due to infection, fatigue or emotion, and how may it be corrected?'[35] The break with the panoptic vision of clinico–pathological medicine was to replace the question: 'Has this patient a disease?' with: 'Is this child growing normally?'[36]

The other component of the increasing visibility of childhood was the gaze over the mind of the developing child. Observation of the mind of the child had arisen earlier in the century in the context of the school medical service, the school psychological service and the emergence of child guidance. Yet it was not until the years of World War II that paediatrics, at the same time as it deployed the survey, also discovered the mind of the child. The Executive Committee of the British Paediatric Association had, in 1943, suggested a close alliance between child guidance clinics and childrens' hospitals when the dangers to children of the war-time situation had risen to such salience.[37] A special Child Psychology Sub-Committee was created in 1944 to examine this area of paediatric practice: it reported in 1946. The Committee argued that paediatricians should show a deeper interest in child psychology because 'it is false to attempt to draw a hard and fast line between physical and psychological disabilities'. Moreover, 'without a study of both the normal and abnormal child, adult neuroses and psychoses cannot be understood'.[38] In 1948 the Child Psychology Sub-Committee pressed for psychiatric departments in all childrens' hospitals.[39]

Thus, in 1953, when Illingworth published the first edition of *The normal child*, he was concerned with describing both physical and psychological normality. For the latter he drew on some American work from the inter-war years carried out by Gesell.[40] Gesell had started charting the behaviour development of normal children from birth to six years old, in 1919, at the Yale Clinic of Child Development (founded in 1911).[41] From this work Gesell created a developmental schedule of 150 items. In 1927 he started on a larger and more comprehensive survey of behaviour development: a relatively homogeneous group of 107 infants were observed, some repeatedly, at 15 age levels from 4 to 56 weeks. In his *Biographies of child development*, of 1939, Gesell extended the growth data on childhood into school life.[42]

For his studies Gesell constructed an observation dome in which the child was placed, while the researchers stood behind a one-way screen. In this 'intimacy of observation with detachment', Gesell, in effect, had devised a structure which followed the principles and architectural outlines of the Panopticon, the chief exception being that the geographical position of observers and observed were reversed.[43] In his writings, too, Gesell implicitly endorsed the mechanisms of surveillance and their disciplinary effects as found in the Panopticon. He predicted, for example, in 1923, that the 'developmental hygiene of the pre-school child will gradually be brought under systematic social control'.[44] And he pointed out in 1939 that too much attention was paid to 'mere training and instruction. Our central task, particularly in the first five years of life, is to discover and to respect individuality.'[45]

In 1965, reflecting on the history of paediatrics, the President of the British Paediatric Association thought it 'fortunate' that 'parallel with paediatric enlightenment ... psychiatry matured'.[46] Fortunate or not, the enlightenment of paediatrics and maturation of psychiatry were both components of the same underlying vision. In post-war paediatrics, the continuous sweep of the survey was united with the observation of childrens' minds. The result was a new paediatrician: the 'new thing was the importance attached to growth, development and adjustment during infancy and childhood. Development was not only physical but also intellectual and social so that behaviour within the family, the school and society had to be included in the wide sweep of his horizons.'[47] If the post-war period 'might be termed the age of the mass survey',[48] it was also the age of the continuous gaze over the normal.

The paediatric principle

In the post-war world, paediatrics was a new discipline with a new vision. It was no longer – as it had been before the war – a specialism: 'paediatrics is in fact general medicine during a particular age period'.[49] A specialist emphasised only one part of a whole whereas paediatrics was concerned with 'the general study of children in health and disease – and is not limited by one aspect of disease or disease of one organ'.[50] Similarly, it was held that children's hospitals were not special hospitals to be classed with urological, ophthalmic, dental and mental hospitals: indeed, it was claimed that children's hospitals were more 'general' than the so-called general hospitals, some of which excluded diseases like pulmonary tuberculosis.[51]

The increasing concern with children 'in health and disease' represented a growing tension between the new discipline and its parent. Until the early years of the national health service, paediatric teaching had begun 'with the assumption that the child is but a miniature version of the adult ... his diseases were the same as in adults but less severe ... his psychological make-up was similar to that of the adult but more innocent ... and that his treatment is identical except that it is scaled down to size'.[52] But, as Apley pointed out a decade or so later, paediatrics was not solely 'diseases of children or medicine in miniature but was a discipline with not only a philosophy but an identity of its own. Childhood can be neither understood nor taught simply by extrapolating back from adults.'[53]

Even as late as 1971, as Mitchell argued, it was 'still sometimes necessary to spell out the different needs of children and adults to specialists in technological medicine who cannot see beyond the organ of their interest'.[54] For example, it was claimed that whereas admission to hospital was usually relatively incidental for the adult, for the child 'it is an experience occurring during a critical period of growth which may leave a lasting mark on his personality'.[55] Thus the British Paediatric Association asserted that the failure to segregate children in accident and emergency departments was not in accord with the generally accepted Report on the Welfare of Children in Hospital, and the Association had also to remind members of the Faculty of Ophthalmologists that their policy of seeing children in ophthalmology departments contravened the Report's recommendations.[56]

If the particular needs of children demanded separate hospitals, they also warranted specialist personnel. The principle of having children in hospital cared for by sick-child nurses was firmly established, the BPA having successfully resisted an attempt by the General Nursing Council to abolish the sick-child nurse register in the early sixties.[57] But 'paediatric' skills were not only needed by nurses; even 'medical technicians and auxiliary workers, who increasingly come into contact with children in hospital, often have no special paediatric training and may be clumsy and inexpert'.[58]

The Report of the Committee on Child Health Services in 1976 (The Court Report)[59] carried the 'paediatric principle' further. It recommended special child-health visitors, general practitioner paediatricians and paediatric experts in various fields of medicine. The Report reaffirmed the view of the BPA[60] that there was a need for paediatric neurologists, cardiologists, nephrologists, endocrinologists, gastro-enterologists, haematologists, and oncologists. Allied specialties included paediatric surgeons, anaesthetists, radiologists, orthopaedic surgeons, ear, nose and throat surgeons, ophthalmologists, dermatologists, medical geneticists, morbid anatomists, histo-pathologists, chemical pathologists, and microbiologists. 'Since paediatric specialists work and share facilities with adult specialists in the same discipline, why are they necessary? The answer is that the needs which justified the separation of paediatrics from adult medicine apply here with equal force.'[61]

Thus 'the childrens' physician metamorphosed into a paediatrician, moved away from his specialisation in organic disease in the age group of birth to puberty, as he realised the importance of development during childhood and infancy'.[62] Growth and development became 'the quintessence of modern paediatrics'[63] and developmental paediatrics the 'foundation' of the discipline.[64] A trend was instituted 'away from pure paediatrics, with its traditional emphasis on diagnosis and treatment of acute medical problems, towards developmental paediatrics'.[65] Capon expressed the prevailing mood in 1950: the various methods of clinical examination, the bulwark of clinical medicine, were 'techniques towards this end ... [but] they must be regarded as preliminaries'.[66]

In extending the survey to the community, paediatrics had invented the normal child. Yet, paradoxically, as Illingworth observed in the preface of his book, 'it is almost impossible to define the normal'.[67] Although the individual child was plotted on a growth and development curve, the implications were somewhat vague: the average was not the normal, those outside the range not necessarily abnormal and maximum growth was not necessarily optimal.[68] Nevertheless, this system of 'non-evaluative' mapping continued and, moreover, became the cornerstone of the new paediatrics. Every child was normal and, at the same time, 'all normal children have behaviour problems'.[69] Notions of normality and abnormality, problems and non-problems lost their discriminatory value. Knowledge of the child became expressed as a single and individual growth trajectory constructed by joining the points marked on a percentile growth chart. Diagnosis and the medical problem, as elements of the Panopticon, were replaced by a constant normalising gaze exercised by a new medical discipline over the growth and development of all children.

7

Disciplines of the survey: 2. psychiatry

In 1924, Newman, the Chief Medical Officer of the Board of Education – and an early exponent of the 'new hygiene' – appointed a Mental Deficiency Committee drawn from the Board of Education and the Board of Control to advise on the problems presented by the mentally defective.[1] The Committee represented the culmination of a series of government moves to identify and provide for mentally defective children.

The Mental Deficiency Act of 1913 had laid upon local education authorities the duty of discovering all the mentally defective children in their areas between the ages of seven and sixteen, and the duty of providing special education for these children was laid down in the Elementary Education (Defective and Epileptic Children) Act of 1914. The local education authority returns on the numbers of mental defectives, however, were extremely variable. Prevalence seemed to vary from 0.73 per 1000 children in one area to 16.14 per 1000 children in another. In the words of the Mental Deficiency Committee: 'It is obvious that no sound administration could be built on such figures, and that little progress could be made until the number of mentally defective children who were likely to be found in any area could be known with reasonable accuracy.'[2] Hence the Mental Deficiency Committee was charged with answering two questions – How many mentally defective children are there? And what is the best thing to do with them?

One of the first decisions of the Committee was that their investigation should not be constrained to children falling within the province of the Board of Education 'but must extend to children of all grades of mental defect.... Any solution of the problem of dealing with one category depended upon, and at the same time affected, the solution of that of dealing with the other category.'[3] The field of enquiry was further extended by taking into consideration mentally defective adults because local mental deficiency authorities also were found to have problems in establishing accurate numbers for those within their jurisdiction.

The Committee decided that the only means of accurately ascertaining the number of mental defectives in the community was by 'intensive investigations in a number of areas'.[4] Six areas were chosen of such varied social and geographical characteristics as to be representative of the country. The particular details of the investigation were handed over to Dr E.O. Lewis who carried out a community survey between 1925 and 1927.[5] Within each area, the mentally defective, and those on the borderline, were identified by a variety of means. School teachers were asked to provide names of those either defective or borderline; those too young to attend school were visited in their own homes, their identities being given by local mental deficiency committees, officers of child welfare clinics, health visitors and district nurses; adult mental defectives were similarly identified by the various institutions, organisations and personnel that worked in and knew the community.

From early in the century when legislation established Dispensary-like mechanisms to monitor the numbers of locations of mental defectives, the local mental deficiency authorities had tried to build up an apparatus of surveillance.[6] It had, however, proved insufficient, and it seemed that many defectives were missed and identification criteria were variable. Lewis's report to the Mental Deficiency Committee was an attempt to remedy these inadequacies. Through a wider network of key community workers, he sought to identify the unknown defective and, by using standardised tests, to make figures from different areas directly comparable. Within this study can be discerned the rudiments of the survey: an apparatus of surveillance to encompass all the community; the community workers (later the survey itself) at the point at which data was gathered; sampling techniques, here used to identify geographical areas for investigation (later used to identify respondents); and standardised criteria by which to discriminate between the normal and abnormal. While Lewis's survey did not attempt to map the normal – as later surveys would – he did examine 'borderline' cases. In particular, he requested teachers, when providing names of the mentally retarded, to list 15% of the most retarded children in each age group so that it was 'almost certain that any child who was really mentally defective appeared in the lists of names of this group'.[7] The true defectives were then identified by group tests and medical examination.

Writing some years later, in 1943, Lemkau and his colleagues, in an international review of statistical studies on the prevalence and incidence of mental disorder in sample populations carried out anywhere in the world, pointed to Lewis's study as a 'model' which no study had emulated. In the meantime there had been other investigations, but these, it was felt, were all flawed in their selection of a sample population.[8]

In Britain in 1934, Slater had published a survey into the incidence of mental disorder because he felt it 'important to form some estimate of mental disorder as a whole' for which there were 'no figures available in

England'.[9] His estimate, however, was based entirely on admission figures from the Board of Control and made no attempt to establish unrecognised morbidity. Slater also published another study (with a similar bias), in 1943, based on admissions to a war-time emergency hospital between 1939 and 1941.[10]

One of the earliest attempts to improve on Lewis's study and estimate the mental health of a total population was the 'mental health survey of a rural area', by Mayer-Gross, published in 1948.[11] The problem, as Mayer-Gross observed, was that surveys in the past had tended only to deal with distinctly abnormal populations. This might have been methodologically advantageous but 'during the last 30 years the interest of psychiatry has shifted from the major psychoses, statistically relatively rare occurrences, to the milder and borderline cases, the minor deviations from the normal average'.[12] It was this new morbidity, more frequent, perhaps more important, of which psychiatry required more knowledge.

The gaze to the 'milder', the 'borderline' and the 'minor deviations' were characteristics of an extended disciplinary apparatus. Mental abnormality began to be seen as not specifically localisable to one person but as a phenomenon which appeared and reappeared in the context of a dynamic and changing 'normal variability'. The new psychiatric gaze was therefore not so much concerned with the examination and celebration of the individual case but with the ever-changing limits of normal variability within the community. Hence the importance of survey techniques which enabled the normal community to be known.

But how was the survey to be adapted for identifying mental disorder? Mayer-Gross was aware of the advantages of surveying everyone within his defined population, but finally decided against it on the grounds that the 'unavoidable publicity would have led to deliberate withholding of cases and facts'.[13] In consequence, he used a modified version of Lewis's technique, starting from local hospital discharges supplemented with information from community workers. Yet there had already been a rigorous community survey of mental health which had encountered little resistance or non-cooperation from respondents: that survey was the government's War-time Social Survey. Glover, the eminent psychoanalyst, hailed the Survey as the beginning of a new social psychiatry. Under the guise of monitoring public opinion, the Survey provided a means of observing national mental health and was therefore 'a ringing blow struck for psychological medicine'.[14]

Glover pointed out that the Social Survey provided 'a comparatively exact instrument for the expression of democratic feeling [and] that it permits the rapid uncovering of avoidable sources of friction ... without denying the social or political significance of public opinion, the Ministry of

Information has established that group feeling is a medico–psychological concern and that it calls for instruments of precision in diagnosis'.[15]

Normalisation of the psychiatric patient

The psychiatric morbidity survey, which was deployed during the war and with increasing frequency in the post-war world, was but one facet of the changing perception of the mentally ill, which, like the similar changes in other areas of medicine, represented a further extension of a disciplinary gaze. In essence, the post-war psychiatric perception was a normalising gaze: not, as in the Panopticon, a normalising gaze over an enclosed and inherently 'abnormal' population, but over an entire domain. This normalising gaze over the whole tended to obliterate the legitimacy of the distinction between normal and abnormal and tended to create one community where before there had been two.

Before and immediately after World War II, two modalities of power can be discerned: on the one hand, the old techniques of confinement, separation and exile of the insane; on the other, the growing strength of a community gaze. The treatment regimens that developed tended to reflect these mechanisms of power. The old principle, that terror and shock were good for the insane (in that it might bridge the gap between the divided communities of sanity and madness), was redeployed in various, though 'humanitarian', forms. The 'emotional shock' of the 1920s,[16] gave way to the shock of insulin coma, the convulsions produced by cardiazol and electro-shock treatment and psychosurgery of the 1930s.[17] En route, thyroidectomy, prolonged narcosis, the production of aseptic meningitis, leucocytosis, controllable fever and high frequency currents were among treatments that had their moments of fashion.[18]

By the 1950s, chemotherapy, earlier discharge and lower rates of hospitalisation had become more common – a process Scull refers to as 'decarceration'.[19] The principle of the 'unlocked door'[20], whereby the old asylum was opened up, was a corollary of a gaze which saw no distinction between healthy and ill, sane and mad. The open door enabled the high walls of the asylum to be pierced: it established the conditions for the emergence of psychiatric day hospitals,[21] regular visiting[22] and treatment regimes which emphasised discharge. Mental institutions could become 'hospitals instead of asylums', emphasis could be placed on 'the clinical needs of the patient and not on his segregation' and fresh terminology could be employed 'free of unhappy associations'.[23]

At the same time as post-war psychiatric policies attempted to end the exclusion of the mentally ill from the community, the boundaries between psychiatric diagnostic categories were challenged. Were the neuroses and psychoses conceptually exclusive? And was the difference between the neuroses and 'normality' qualitative? Inter-war psychiatry had been largely divided into those who managed the neuroses in the community – the special clinics, out-patients, the GP surgery – and those who guarded over the psychoses within the mental hospital. The post-war world saw a unified psychiatry which dealt with both neuroses and psychoses: the old hospital psychiatry 'absorbed not only the principles of psychotherapy but also its practitioners'.[24]

At the same time, psychiatry took over from the neurologists the little that the latter continued to claim of the neuroses. Walshe had grudgingly accepted a chapter on psychoneurosis in his *Diseases of the nervous system*, of 1940, but, by the fifth edition of 1947, their inclusion was only justified to the extent that they had to be separated from neurological problems in the diagnosis. In the eighth edition, of 1955, the chapter had been rewritten and restricted itself solely to 'problems the neurologists alone can usefully undertake'.[25] Brain's *Diseases of the nervous system*, first published in 1933, at first reflected Brain's belief that mind and brain should be kept together;[26] but, in 1951, neurasthenia was dropped and anxiety neurosis followed suit in 1962.[27] In effect, the attempt during the war to create a unified neuro-psychiatry[28] had failed.

Whereas before the war, separation into those who treated psychoses and those who treated neuroses had been usual, after the war, the assumption was that they were united and the 'constant danger' was that they might be sub-divided.[29] Similarly, the cognitive and clinical separation of the psychoses from the neuroses appeared to be increasingly problematic. In 1965 Merskey & Tonge in their text, *Psychiatric illness*, suggested it was difficult to distinguish between psychoses and neuroses.[30] In 1970 Howells proposed a new psychiatric nosology which would integrate the psychoses and the neuroses.[31] Crown, in his *Essential principles of psychiatry*, of 1970, suggested that all psychiatric phenomena were quantitative and not qualitative deviations from normal.[32] On the other hand, Hamilton argued in *Clinical psychopathology*, of 1974, that the psychoses were 'true illnesses in which a sharp break in the personality occurs'.[33] Trethowan perhaps best summed up the mood in his *Psychiatry*, of 1979, when he claimed that the question of how far psychoses differ qualitatively from abnormal emotional reactions 'still remains one of psychiatry's fundamental problems'.[34]

The Memorandum on the Future Organisation of Psychiatric Services, in 1945, had commented that 'where psychiatry begins and ends has not been settled'.[35] The boundary between the normal population and the neuroses was ill defined. 'The psychological disorders in these conditions are mainly quantitative exaggerations of normal psychological features, so it is often difficult to decide where normality ends and abnormality begins.' Indeed, it was possible to argue that these mental problems were 'not illnesses in the usual sense of the word'.[36]

This blurring of the distinction between the normal and the abnormal was considerably aided by the findings of the new surveys (which were themselves, of course, part of the new perception). Results from the large American community studies of psychiatric morbidity, commenced immediately after the war, were being published and they recorded extremely high prevalence rates for the neuroses.[37] Studies by Primrose, and later by Brown, confirmed the wide distribution of psychiatric morbidity.[38] Various surveys of morbidity within the community or within general practice consultations offered further support[39] and the writings of Michael Balint led to the intrusion of a 'psychiatric' perspective into all consultations.[40]

It was found, for example, that between 30 and 90% of the 'organic' complaints under the care of general clinicians had a psychiatric component.[41] Psychiatry could therefore intrude into the very practice of medicine itself, observing, checking, correcting, monitoring. 'The nature of our speciality makes us especially conscious of the psychological and social problems caused by illness.'[42] Psychiatrists would, of necessity, have to teach human relations or those psychological processes which were vital for the practice of medicine.[43] The importance of this claim had been presented to the House of Commons in the call for a Royal Commission on Medical Education in 1961[44] and the report of the Commission in 1968 had commended this perspective and stressed the role of psychiatry in understanding the very essence of practice and the fullest comprehension of patient problems.[45]

From the first edition of their book, *A textbook of psychiatry*, in 1927, Henderson & Gillespie had included a brief historical review of the subject which ended with the ' Hospital period'. In 1944, in recognition of the new domain of psychiatry, they added a section on the 'Social or community period'. Here they recommended the extension of psychiatry into the community: in the education of those in charge of nurseries, residential schools, and hostels, in the selection and education of youth leaders and into industry and the field of sickness absence. 'It seems best that psychiatry should extend to the community in these ways, where the ground is already explored and known, before it tries to extend still further and become part of community life, of government and even of international relations.'[46]

The fabrication of subjects

In 1911, in his book *Unsoundness of mind*, Clouston pointed out that neurasthenia was sometimes seen among highly educated young women, though it was uncommon among healthily reared young country women. From this he concluded that 'if men and women live as they should do [neurasthenia] would scarcely exist at all'.[47] In 1937, Ross, in his *The common neuroses*, claimed that the neuroses were caused by a faulty response to life's difficulties.[48]

These two diagnoses differed considerably in form from insanity. The insane were exiled for being mad in a community of sanity; the effect of this policy of exclusion was to reaffirm the rationality of the 'normal' community. Neurasthenia and, more important, the later neuroses, operated by a different mechanism. In these cases the identification of the disorder had positive effects: the patients could change and be made well, and appropriate life styles and relationships could be indicated to the general population. Thus, whereas madness had reaffirmed through negative action (exclusion), the neuroses both reaffirmed and effected change through positive action (surveillance). The invention of the neuroses, therefore, constituted a lighter more subtle discipline and, at the same time, one with multiple effects: where madness had merely reaffirmed, by comparison, one aspect of mental functioning, the neuroses could potentially create its multi-dimensional totality.

Panoptic power had fabricated bodies by making them the objects of an observing eye. The new regime exercised surveillance over the whole population and, because it observed the mind of everyone, was in a better position to make the individual a point of articulation for power: both an effect of power and a point from which power was exercised. Where the Panopticon had created individuals as objects the extended community gaze established an analysable social space, around and between these same bodies, which came to be seen as one of their essential characteristics. In other words, the gaze began to fabricate a subjective space around the object of the body. Such a change in the effects of the psychiatric gaze is in evidence from late in the inter-war period when the psychiatric patient made an appearance as a part of the treatment regime instead of its object.

The mental hospital began to change from a place of exile to a point of rehabilitation. From a regime which repressed and negated, by the bluntness of its powers of exclusion and containment, emerged a disciplinary machine which segmented and ordered hierarchically so that the mentally ill might become part of the machinery of power rather than a victim of it. The mental hospital was not simply an institution of exclusion; instead, its characteristics, its structures, its darkest, remotest parts could be analysed, respatialised and integrated to create a total environment, a subtle disciplinary machine.

The patient was no longer the object of the hospital but the subject of its essence. The patient was no longer a member of the community of the insane but an individual with 'a biography, a social setting, a constitution, with experiences undergone and effects rendered, a life with purpose and with handicaps'. Treatment, 'like the illnesses themselves must be viewed as a whole scheme or pattern of activity': it 'starts from the moment of introduction to the patient'.[49] Thereafter, the social organisation of the hospital could provide a total therapeutic regime. Improved communication enabled problems of meaning, of handling knowledge, of reaching consensus on goals, etc., to be debated and analysed throughout the hospital hierarchy (and ultimately to lead to the demise of the latter).[50] The integration of administration and therapy could, in effect, make administrative action – which for so long had acted as an impediment – a therapy in its own right.[51] The vision emerged of a therapeutic community which would act on the patient in a multiplicity of ways.

With this view of the hospital as a therapy in itself (not merely a place of therapy), its various effects could be analysed. Its internal arrangements were increasingly reorganised to generate the sort of environment which would enable the patient to be returned to the community.[52] Yet the hospital with a power for positive effect could also be construed, with inappropriate organisation, as a power for negative effect. Might not the hospital be creating some of the problems it was meant to be treating? A new analysis of space, routine and organisation emerged in the 1950s, which stressed the negative effects of the hospital. A new discourse on labelling, stigma and institutionalisation arose both in medicine and in the related social sciences:[53] a discourse which opposed the depersonalising aspects of institutional life (which had been one of the chief mechanisms of the Panopticon) and replaced it with notions of personal identity and subjectivity.

The importance accorded patient meaning and subjectivity within the new mechanisms of power meant that, at the very moment of its triumph, psychiatry had to discard the external referrents by which patients had previously been judged and objectified. The problem with the promotion of mental health, Sir Aubrey Lewis observed in 1958, was that it had 'no operational referrents' and it could only be expressed in terms 'undefined and undefinable'.[54] Psychiatry had to proceed with caution. MacCalman, as early as 1949, advised his colleagues to 'resist the implied flattery of being consulted about ever wider social and national problems'.[55] As Curran argued in his Presidential Address to the Section of Psychiatry of the Royal Society of Medicine a few years later, psychiatry had to resist expansionist claims.[56]

This position was mirrored in the human sciences, which, from the same period onwards, developed an 'anti-psychiatry' whose main focus of attack was the apparently arbitrary referrents by which psychiatrists judged their patients.[57] Yet even as these critics decried the visible excess of a psychiatry with 'objective' referrents, changes in the form and mechanism of the psychiatric gaze were already under way to make its operation more invisible and more pervasive.

The relationship between psychiatrist and patient began to be reconstrued. The disciplinary gaze, which sought to encompass the totality of the patient, in a self-reflexive gesture, also turned to examine the psychiatrist. Besides listening to and observing the patient, the doctor had to be self-aware:[58] 'What is my attitude? Am I understanding the situation from the patient's point of view, or from mine alone? What is my reaction to his behaviour?'[59] In short, the interview had to examine both the patient's and the psychiatrist's words and actions. 'Thus in an interview there are at least two persons to be heard and two to be observed both as individuals and in terms of their interaction.'[60] Both psychiatrists and patients were subjects.

The diagnosis, as classically understood, began to disappear. For some, it was replaced by the 'formulation – a construction of working hypotheses of the nature of the patient's problem'[61] – for others, a 'multi-dimensional diagnosis'.[62] In effect, these new diagnostic conventions represented an attempt to summarise what was individual about the patient. Thus psychiatry moved from classification to individual description: 'the most essential feature in the recent development of psychiatry has been that the diagnosis of disease has given place to absorption in the personal tragedy of individuals'.[63] It was probably no coincidence that a phenomenological influence spread through psychiatry in the 1960s.[64]

Under the old regime the psychiatric judgement of normality or abnormality had been a function of external criteria; now the patient began to become his or her own judge and referrent. 'Is the present state foreign to the patient's previous personality?' was the first question to be posed.[65] Or, put another way, 'the most important comparison is probably that between the present state and the previous personality'.[66] A technology of 'coping' was theoretically refined and a vast literature on 'stress' emerged in the post-war years. Patients would define their own limits and make their own decisions: 'when a patient calls on his doctor for help he generally implies that his own efforts are not enough'.[67]

A psychiatry based on the external referrent of the psychiatrist objectified the patient: a psychiatry which defined the patient as a subject, which explored and valued subjectivity, signified a new power. When the psychiatrist could freely enter the mind of the patient, when the patient internalised the criteria of normality and became his own judge, then the power of the new surveillance could move with greater speed, but above all with invisibility. A liberated and humane psychiatry, together with the concerned human sciences, could be crystallised around an efficient and pervasive gaze which analysed and fabricated the mind of the subject.

8

Disciplines of the survey: 3. general practice

The changes in medicine which occurred at the end of the eighteenth century ushered in a new 'regime of truth' in which the deepest secrets of the human body could only be revealed by a detailed examination and analysis.[1] Consequently, the history of medicine from that period is also the history of a reductionist gaze to the body of the patient, characterised by a growth in the number of hospitals, the invention of more investigative procedures, and the emergence of a specialised division of labour within the medical profession which enabled the clinical gaze to become more detailed.

The process of investigating and examining bodies grew significantly in the twentieth century. First, there was a rapid growth in the number of hospital beds: between 1911 and 1938, for example, the number of beds in voluntary hospitals doubled.[2] By 1929, when the Local Government Act placed the old Poor Law hospitals under local authority control, the *Lancet* claimed that 'the centre of gravity of medicine [has] shifted from the home to the hospital and clinic' and this would have 'the effect of popularising hospitals still further'.[3]

Second, the process of diagnosis within hospitals, the 'gaze' which delineated the outline of the body of the patient, was considerably enhanced by the emergence of complex laboratory-based investigations. Such was the growth of these new diagnostic facilities in the inter-war years that a new specialty of clinical pathology (which was later to sub-divide further into morbid anatomy, clinical chemistry, haematology and bacteriology) emerged.[4]

The growth of hospitals to enclose bodies and the development of laboratory tests to analyse them was accompanied by further specialisation as different parts of the body were separately investigated. Specialisation – as a reflection of the 'natural' structure of the body of the patient – was itself seen as an inherently 'natural' process: 'With the growth of knowledge and the development of technique the mastery of all medicine by one man became impossible and division of labour naturally followed.'[5]

One effect of the strengthening of the panoptic vision in the inter-war years was the undermining of general practice. True, the GP was employed in the examination and investigation of individual bodies but the hospital setting, with its accompanying resources, produced a more efficient and powerful gaze. The GP might have been trained in a panoptic structure (the hospital) and be cognisant with the analytic principles of the panoptic vision, but the conditions of general practice – particularly a widely dispersed patient population – ensured that the gaze was less effective, less penetrating, when compared with hospital practice.

The growth in numbers of hospital beds did little therefore to help general practice – indeed, at times, the GP was specifically excluded. Lord Moynihan, the eminent surgeon, advised against putting local GPs on the staffs of the new municipal hospitals unless they had 'proper credentials'.[6] The advent of the national health service in 1948 further promoted this separation by forcing doctors to choose between a hospital career or one in general practice. The NHS, claimed the *British Medical Journal* with some exaggeration, created divisions where none had existed before.[7]

Access to the new laboratory-based diagnostic techniques remained under the control of hospital specialists; and GPs, until the 1950s and 1960s, were not allowed to use them. The GP was therefore seen to be in different circumstances from the hospital specialist 'who can try out a new remedy extensively and have controls' and who had access to the laboratory as 'a final court of appeal'.[8] The growth of specialisation further undermined the status of the GP. 'Early specialisation is forced upon us by the growth of knowledge and the limit of human life.'[9] GPs were, of necessity, excluded from this process as it was impossible for 'any but exceptional men to keep an up-to-date knowledge of more than a few of the special branches of medicine'.[10] Indeed, it was suggested in 1926 that general practice might disappear altogether under the weight of specialisms.[11]

By 1938 the *British Medical Journal* was aware that an atmosphere 'unfavourable and detrimental to the status of general practice created in medical schools was not a new thing' and, indeed, in the same year the President of the BMA pointed out that 'there is a tendency for this branch of the profession to sink lower and lower in the estimation both of the public and of the student body from which the profession itself is recruited'.[12] A correspondent of the *British Medical Journal* objected to the GP being described as the backbone of the profession, as it suggested the absence of a brain.[13]

Yet, at the same time as the status of general practice was so much in decline, an alternative vision of clinical practice was coming into focus. It began to be realised that only in general practice could the temporal elements of illness be plotted. 'It is only the family doctor who can follow the history of individuals during 30 or 40 years, summing up the hereditary and prenatal influences, the effects of wrong habits in childhood, the final results of infantile and youthful ailments and the first causes of premature decay or death.'[14] The GP was, moreover, in a position to superimpose on this temporal dimension of the natural history of illness – its regressions, disappearances, appearances and exacerbations – the grid formed by the intimacies of social relationships.

In the inter-war years these two strands of an emergent community gaze were realised in the now classic work of MacKenzie in Scotland and Pickles in Wensleydale. From his general practice in Aberdeen, MacKenzie made meticulous studies of 'ordinary' diseases and their changes over time.[15] In Wensleydale, Pickles added to this by recording, over a number of years, the location, distribution, spread and timing of various epidemic diseases, particularly in the context of his patients' relationships and interactions: the result was a social mapping of his general practice community.[16] For example, he was able to plot the various contacts, casual and intimate, of a young girl with hepatitis who, despite Pickles's advice, had left her sick-bed and visited a local fair.[17]

While MacKenzie and Pickles were busy constructing the analytical lines which would enable the social body to be mapped and defined, other GPs concentrated on the details and intimacies of the patient's social localisation. Throughout the inter-war years, Brackenbury, the Secretary of the BMA, advocated a 'social worker' role for the GP.[18] Many GPs expressed interest in the newly emerging psychotherapeutic skills and reported using them with their patients.[19] Lindsay, the President of the British Medical Association, in 1938 argued that a role in mental hygiene might stop the declining status of the GP. It was the GPs who could 'lead the attack' on the large amounts of major and minor functional nervous disease in the community and for this role they would require instruction in the principles of medical psychology.[20] It was this perspective that the *British Medical Journal* endorsed when it suggested, in 1938, that the future of general practice was in the 'early recognition of disease states, the application in ordinary cases of those psychotherapeutic methods which are becoming more and more a national need, the proper coordination of extending specialist services, and the more effective education of the public in medical and health matters'.[21]

Surveys of sickness

The Peckham health centre had ensured that the morbidity within its population was measured during the 1930s and the Government Survey of Sickness, from 1944, as part of the War-time Social Survey, had kept a constant check on the amount of illness in the community. The results of the latter were summarised by Stocks in *Sickness in the population of England and Wales: 1944–47*, published in 1949.[22]

After the war further surveys of morbidity were carried out. In 1949 Pemberton recorded the age, sex and diagnosis of all people consulting eight general practices in Sheffield during one week in winter and a week in summer.[23] McGregor carried out a similar survey of his own practice in Scotland, in 1950[24] and Fry published his analysis of a year's morbidity in his practice in south-east London, in 1952.[25] Prior to these surveys, GPs had not measured morbidity in the communities they served. Was it mere coincidence that a group of GPs, after the war, thought it important to measure and publish their findings on community morbidity at the same time as the survey was mapping other areas of the social body? Or was it that, prior to these surveys, the GP could not measure community morbidity because it had not been conceptualised as such?

In his book, *The structure of scientific revolutions*, Kuhn points out that when chemical compounds were seen as mixtures, the measurement of the relative proportions of different elements comprising the compounds, while technically feasible, was seen as valueless. A theory of mixtures would claim that, on measurement, any ratio of elements might be found so there seemed little point in identifying exact ratios from an infinite number of possibilities. But when compounds were seen as chemical combinations of fixed proportions of elements, the analysis of ratios of elements in a compound became of vital importance. In short, a theory of mixtures, in its basic assumptions, had ensured that certain measurements, though technically feasible, were never made; a new theory with a different set of assumptions made the same measurement of crucial significance.[26]

In the same way, the rapid measurement of a phenomenon in general practice, which until then had remained unmeasured, suggests a shift of perspective. Prior to the survey, morbidity existed in patients who were analysed and treated individually and while the addition of these individual cases was possible it served little purpose. The survey, on the other hand, established a perception of the community as something inherently measurable and calculable: the survey was part of a new 'regime of truth' which, in its focus on the social rather than the individual body, introduced a new direction and imperative in medical investigation.

The surveyors themselves partly justified their studies on the needs of future planning in the NHS (itself a structure which embraced the community), but principally on the need to know something of the nature of the more common diseases. As Fry argued, it was only through such surveys of GP records or from national morbidity surveys that it was possible to 'uncover the extent and form of the vast amount of minor ill-health in the community'.[27] Thus, from a general medicine which examined grossly deranged bodies with their localised lesions, within a panoptic structure, general practice began to turn its gaze to the minor, the transient, the constantly moving illnesses which traversed the social body.

In 1953, Logan, the Chief Medical Statistician at the General Register Office, published an analysis of the clinical records of eight general practices during the period April 1951 to March 1952.[28] A report of the Statistics Sub-Committee of the Registrar-General's Advisory Committee on Medical Nomenclature and Statistics, entitled *The measurement of morbidity*, was published in 1954[29] and an overview of the findings of *The survey of sickness 1943–1952*, by Logan & Brooke, was published in 1957.[30] In 1955, 106 GPs drawn from the Research Register of the College of General Practitioners agreed to record all morbidity in their practices between May 1955 and April 1956 for Logan and Cushion of the General Register Office. The results were published in 1958.[31]

This latter Morbidity Survey – the first major project undertaken by the newly founded College for General Practitioners – seemed to strike a chord for many GPs: 'The habit of recording soon grew upon [the doctors taking part in the Survey] and a curious sense of incompleteness was felt when the extra records were no longer needed. The habit was so entrenched in some practices that recording was kept up, using the same methods, long after the survey year came to an end.'[32] Just as the imperative of the Panopticon was to analyse individual bodies, a new perception began to command the surveillance of the social body. The Survey established, in the words of the College journal, 'a new method of observational research which has undoubtedly come to stay'.[33]

The College of General Practitioners formed an Epidemic Observation Unit, which, like the studies of Pickles, studied the changing distribution of various diseases in the community.[34] A College Records Unit was proposed to pursue 'the continued study of total morbidity'.[35] Regional faculties of the College, when urged to produce some research, carried out surveys: the South-East England Faculty published its report on epidemic winter vomiting in 1955[36] the South-West Faculty, a survey of GP obstetric cases;[37] and the Yorkshire Faculty, a survey of unrecorded cases of cancer in 1956.[38]

Finlay surveyed morbidity in six practices, in 1954[39] Horder & Horder examined 2000 first-time consultations, in 1954[40] Fry completed a five-year study of his practice morbidity, in 1956;[41] Backett and his co-workers described the diagnoses made in a practice of 3000 in one year;[42] Crombie surveyed his own practice, in 1957;[43] Theakston carried out a 'social survey' of his country practice during six months of 1956;[44] in 1959 Handfield-Jones reported on one year's work in general practice,[45] Bancroft, on a survey of patients with chronic illness in a general practice,[46] and Crombie, on a casualty survey.[47] Within a few years the survey was being used to examine many facets of general practice and in so doing transformed its cognitive base.

The technology of the survey potentially enabled post-war general practice to monitor the community over time and to map its distributions over space. It became possible to envisage that the very earliest manifestations of disease in the community might be identified: the GP for instance was 'undoubtedly in an ideal situation to make useful observation and valuable records of 'the very earliest phases of stress disorders and psychiatric illness'.[48] It also became apparent that 'continuity of observation is one of the advantages of general practice'[49] – continuity over time, over diseases, over patients and over social networks.

With the gradual extension of the survey and the increasing deployment of the community disciplinary gaze in the post-war world, an outline of a respatialised medicine began to emerge; a new map came into focus on which could be plotted new diseases, practices, effects and specialties. At the point where a concern with childhood intersected various techniques for the observation of normal children, a new paediatrics emerged; at another point there was a new configuration in the field of mental illness from where a revitalised psychiatry crystallised out its new shape and concerns. Similarly, at the point where the survey, which uncovered 'ordinary' diseases, and the imperatives of continuous community observation came together, the conditions were created for a new general practice to be formed. These realignments in the broad field of medicine in the community did not occur instantly – and, indeed, are far from accomplished to the present day – but in the early post-war years the possibility of an alternative form of practice, a transformed problematic, a new gaze, began to be felt in the traditional domain of the GP. New 'conditions of possibility', to use Foucault's phrase, began to influence the production of a new discourse in general practice which, in its turn, began to have various effects on social and institutional practices.[50]

Thus, in the post-war world, prevention of disease from its earliest appearances, and continuity of care, became an important claim of the new general practice. The British Medical Association report on *General practice and the training of the GP*, published in 1950, defined the GP's role in terms of continuous and preventive care and health education and concluded that general practice 'has as its goal the study of the whole man'.[51] Continuity of care and preventive medicine were identified by the Report of the General Practice Steering Committee, of 1952 (which proposed a College of General Practitioners), as 'unique, positive features' in the role of the family doctor who had previously been defined in essentially negative terms as a non-specialist.[52]

The other great discovery (and creation) of the survey in general practice was the almost limitless domain of the normal and the range of normal variation. Before the war the GP's function could be seen as 'cure' as in the hospital; during the war it was to maintain 'fitness and efficiency'; after the war the GP was faced by 'a mass of apparently unexplained sickness, much of it undiagnosable and much of it self-limiting'.[53] Post-war general practice developed an extensive discourse on the normal and its variation which manifested itself in a variety of often seemingly contradictory positions.

First, there were those GPs who wanted to use the survey as an instrument for prising apart the apparent continuity between illness and normality. Pinsent couched the problem in terms of distinguishing the trivial from the normal. 'Only by observing the course of diseases and their natural history can we learn the full significance of each departure from normal.'[54] Furthermore, through the survey, it would be possible to establish the order and frequency of illness in the community which could then be used as a reference point.[55]

The need to separate the normal, the trivial and 'real' illness also underpinned the arguments of those in general practice who, throughout the 1950s and 1960s, complained that general practice was being overwhelmed by 'trivia'. Over-use of services for trivial complaints was commonly believed to be general;[56] patients were seen to demand services 'if their minor symptoms have not subsided in ten days';[57] the GP was thought to have been reduced to a 'mere signpost and disher-out of placebos'.[58]

This new discourse on the extent of minor and trivial illness, which came to preoccupy much of the general practice literature during the 1950s, also found expression in the proposed rejection of traditional medical diagnostic categories so as to enable these new phenomena to be measured. An editorial, in 1955, in the College of General Practitioners' *Research Newsletter* argued 'might not we GPs accept the fact that health is a state in which variations from the normal or average may occur without disease necessarily being present?'[59] GPs who attempted to measure morbidity in their practices, increasingly found themselves accepting the seeking of medical advice[60] or 'spells of sickness' as the criteria of morbidity.[61] In effect, patient-based criteria began to replace nosological referrents in the identification of illness.

Another element in the perception of the new general practice, which the survey engendered, was the final conflation of normality and abnormality. This first presented as a methodological problem. It was found – so it was claimed – that in the Survey of Sickness, under intense questioning, 'most people could be got to confess to some minor complaint'.[62] The methodological problem, however, was rapidly transposed into a conceptual one:

might not symptoms, as the Peckham health centre discovered, be widespread in the community? Might not those who failed to consult the GP be equally as ill as those who choose to seek his advice? Was the so-called normal, truly healthy, or did the normal move in and out of illnesses in the community beyond the immediate clinical gaze? Were the findings of the Survey of Sickness methodological artefacts or did they represent a correct view of 'normal' health?

In their survey of 2000 first-time consultations, carried out in 1953, Horder & Horder also visited 98 randomly selected families and noted their morbidity. It seemed from these findings that perhaps two-thirds of patients' illnesses went unreported to the GP. Horder & Horder commented: 'This result may seem a little difficult to believe.'[63] Yet this discovery was supported by Backett who, in his survey of 16 000 consultations, also arranged for a random sample of 101 families to be visited for six months by social workers to record their morbidity.[64]

In parallel, particularly under the influence of American research, medical sociology discovered 'illness behaviour'.[65] Surveys were carried out, often with doctors, of the perception of illness and use of services in the community.[66] Symptoms and illness were found to be relatively common occurrences and use of services unrelated to severity. A recurrent problem with these studies was the interpretation to be placed on the apparent variability in reporting of symptoms, according to period of recall, mood, context, etc. At first, these problems were treated as methodological in nature – something essentially to be overcome to establish 'true' morbidity; later, they were interpreted as signifying the very essence of the non-localisable, shifting, transient symptomatology which both defined and characterised the social body.[67]

The psycho–social context

The survey established morbidity as an ephemeral point at which patient characteristics, relationships and context manifested themselves. It also focused medical attention on those very peculiarities of the social body which brought morbidity – especially the minor and trivial – into, albeit brief, relief.

The newly formed Section of General Practice at the Royal Society of Medicine held a discussion on 'What is general practice?', in 1950. It was argued that 'the essence of general practice is to live amongst your patients as a definite cog in the whole machine, knowing them so well both in health and in sickness, and from birth until death'. The new 'discovery' of social medicine as human ecology was commended as showing that there was more to medicine than hospital practice. If the GP was to know properly and treat his patients then the patient's 'parents, his family life, his home, his work, his tastes, his recreations' must be studied. Within this context, all problems thrown up by the interaction, transitory and enduring, of movements within the social body, were of concern to the GP: 'I believe there is no case, however trivial, which is completely without interest.'[68]

The discourse on trivia, which emerged during the 1950s, in general practice, was partly a consequence of the survey, which had discovered illness to be ubiquitous. Trivia was also, however, the point on which the new clinical gaze to the psycho–social was articulated. The discourse on trivia was therefore the product of two elements of the surveillance apparatus: the survey itself, which mapped the social body, and the gaze to the relationships within that body. 'In a study of the natural history of disease, especially where emotions are concerned, it is important to study the patient against this home background and in his natural environment.'[69]

The survey had shown certain forms of illness to be intimately related to the social body (which therefore constituted its points of reference). Similarly, the new 'psychological' gaze rejected illness as an external entity, a neurological abstraction which invaded the patient's body; rather, it was an expression of the patient's biography. 'Where the purpose of illness is important in the patient's life-scheme, attempts to remove it will be in vain or even "hazardous".'[70] The patient's 'medical history is only a part of the story, and to consider it alone – as we used to do in the past – is to practise what the late Dr. Crookshank called Farm-Yard Medicine'.[71]

During the 1950s, therefore, a reconstruction began to take place in aspects of the GP's role. The importance of the GP as friend, guide and counsellor was continually stressed;[72] the history of general practice was so constructed to promote a vision of a distant era in which 'deep insight into family life and character' constituted the essence of a well-regarded general practice.[73] Emotional illness, stress and psychotherapy, it was argued, were integral elements of any general practice.[74]

This analysis of the work of the GP found its full theoretical expression in the work of Balint, published in the 1950s.[75] Balint argued that the medical gaze in general practice should not be directed to the interior of the body but outwards to the patient's ever-changing social context. The function of the doctor was to listen and form a relationship – not with a passive object but with a patient as subject. The examination of the psycho–social thus functioned as a mechanism for seeing and treating the patient as a subject. The discovery of the 'relationship' between doctor and patient and the importance assigned to it, assumed a coming together of subjects whose behaviour and attitudes would mutually affect one another.[76]

Moreover, the reasons for visiting the doctor were reconstrued in terms of 'unorganised illness' which required ordering. The whole configuration of illness, patient, and doctor was therefore rearranged, and from it emerged the 'problem' of trivia and the gaze to the subjective patient since it was the patient's meanings, decisions and subjective world which triggered the decision to consult rather than the dictates of a localised, organic pathology. As Horder claimed, several years later, when describing the influence of Balint, 'since each patient is unique, diagnosis must be like biography and is inseparable from treatment'.[77]

The organisation of general practice

The new extended clinical gaze embodied a perception which reconstrued various aspects of illness – its nature, its forms, its temporal orderings and its distributions; it enabled illness to be seen in terms of the incessant movements within a social space and thereby brought about a reassessment of the identity of the patient. But it was also a mechanism, a particular technology, for both creating and monitoring these new phenomena. Thus the survey emerged as both a component of, and means of realising, a community disciplinary apparatus, and the consequent constant gaze over the population found its expression in the emergence of new institutional arrangements in general practice.

As a mechanism for monitoring the community, the gaze had to examine 'normal' people, it had to map social relationships and illness distributions, it had to extend itself physically from a medical-centre to a community-periphery. Health centres provided one element of this structure. Health centres had been proposed by the Dawson Report of 1920 as points of coordination between hospital and community and as the base for domiciliary services.[78] The Peckham health centre – though in many ways eccentric – had realised some of these proposals and the National Health Service Act, of 1964, suggested further extension of the health centre ideal.[79]

In the event, it was to be almost two decades before health centres became widespread; only a handful existed during the 1950s though it was alleged that in these, when they were successful, a 'spirit of enterprise and the "new look" in social medicine dominate the scene'.[80] The delay in establishing health centres was mainly due to resistance by GPs. A postal survey by the British Medical Association, in 1951, discovered only 38% of GPs supported health centres; yet a few years earlier, during the war, a majority of GPs had declared themselves in favour in a similar survey.[81]

The effect of the war on GP perception was important. The war had imposed a panoptic structure on the whole community in terms of a constancy of surveillance and monitoring. The survey had emerged during the war as an instrument of observation; the emergency health service had, for the first time in Britain, offered a comprehensive health care system to the whole of the population. Within this integrated community the idea of a health centre could therefore be seen positively, as an institutional arrangement which might further these various processes of mapping and maintaining the social body. Within the armed forces, on the other hand, with even closer integration and more pervasive surveillance and disciplinary mechanisms, support for health centres was even more enthusiastic: of doctors serving in the armed forces, 83% voted in favour of returning to health centres.[82]

When the war was over and the disciplinary machine which had embraced a whole society was relaxed, the appeal of health centres diminished. It was only with the more gradual extension of generalised surveillance techniques into general practice during the 1950s (in terms of the survey and the psycho–social gaze), and the removal of financial impediments in the 1960s, that the health centre could once more be seen as an ideal institutional mechanism through which to deliver good general practice.[83]

Health centres, when they came to be built, enabled various elements of a Dispensary-like apparatus to be institutionalised. First, they offered the opportunity for integrating all community medical services. They enabled, for example, local authority clinics – some of the original manifestations of the Dispensary – to be integrated with general practice. Thus Edwards reported child health clinics, school clinics and family planning clinics within health centres in Devon.[84] Second, health centres made special provision for certain essentially 'normal' population groups, perhaps a retirement clinic, an obesity clinic, a motherhood clinic and, more specifically, for clinics to be devoted entirely to screening and surveillance, for example diabetes clinics and hypertension clinics. Finally, the health centre provided a base and point of communication for the growing 'health care team' which, particularly in its community role, enabled medical observation to be further extended.

The general practice 'health care team' was an invention of this same era. In the late 1950s and early 1960s there were less than twenty 'attached' health visitors, district nurses and midwives in the whole country.[85] More attachment schemes were advocated by the Gillie Report of 1963.[86] By the beginning of 1969, 25% of district nurses, 29% of health visitors and 15% of midwives employed by the local authority were working in attachment schemes (in all, several thousand paramedical staff being involved).[87]

The Gillie Report saw the functions of the GP as threefold: as a 'first-line defence' in the health service, as an intermediary between patient and specialist, and for mobilising and coordinating health and welfare services. It was particularly in respect of this latter function that Gillie believed that attachment schemes would be beneficial. 'The borderline between medicine and social science lies in general practice', and it was as an aid to managing this area of preventive care, personal relationships and public health, that nurses, health visitors and midwives would be invaluable.[88] The need for further 'ancillary help' formed a central plank in the struggle over the GP's Charter in 1965[89] and, as attachment schemes became more common, so the health care team became the normal context of general practice work. Drury, after a year as Nuffield Travelling Fellow in general practice, concluded 'This concept of the future pattern of general practice in Great Britain is widely accepted.'[90]

The health care team, however, did not usurp GPs' functions – as it was at first feared – but extended their range. As Fry argued 'nurses and health visitors working with general practitioners increase the scope of their work but this increase is not through delegation or dilution of the responsibility of the doctor'.[91] They would work, like the GP, with the 'common diseases of the community'. The nurse could become involved in screening and diagnostic procedures, the health visitor, as the medical social worker of the practice, could be the 'contact girl' with other services and its activist in the social, preventive and educational aspects of medical care and welfare.[92]

The health centre and the health care team were components in a network of surveillance that discovered, identified and monitored the common disease, the minor symptom, the transient illness which hardly marked the body of the patient. The trivial became important, not because it suddenly appeared and apparently threatened the very existence of general practice, but because it was born at the point of intersection of various lines of force which now traversed the conceptual, social and institutional domains of medicine.

The survey both discovered the trivial and also enabled it to be explored, particularly its distributions, both spatially and temporally. The psycho-social gaze, which sought to encompass the intimacies of social relationships, came to rest especially on patient problems in which particular localised, organic pathologies were absent. The replacement of the norm by the normal threw into relief the problem of trivia as an instance of normal variation. The changing institutional arrangements of general practice enabled the trivial to be encompassed in relation to buildings, in the context of special clinics, and by the extended medical arm of the health care team. General practice was in a position to desert the detailed, reductionist analyses of the Panopticon and to turn its gaze to the casual movements and the brief appearances of illnesses within a social body.

9

Disciplines of the survey: 4. geriatrics

Geriatrics was a specialty born directly of the survey. Its first stirrings were in 1935 when Warren surveyed the morbidity among older patients in an old Poor Law infirmary;[1] but as a subject with a specific identity it can probably be dated to Sheldon's classic survey, of 1948.[2] It was the latter survey, together with similar surveys in the following years, which established the outline of a new discipline and at the same time constituted the basis of its cognitive framework.

In 1944, the Nuffield Foundation had sponsored a survey of old age under Seebohm Rowntree. Published in 1947, this survey examined old peoples' incomes, housing, living conditions, recreation, employment, etc.[3] Investigation of the medical condition of old people, however, was entrusted to Sheldon, a hospital physician in Wolverhampton. Sheldon took a random sample of 1 in 30 old people living in Wolverhampton – in all some 583 people – visited their homes, recorded their living conditions and relationships and made an impression of their physical state. The result was the first record of the health of a normal community of the aged. 'It is hoped that this short description of some of the physical and social problems connected with old age may bring home the fact that this is a branch of medicine in which simple, direct observation can still pay an ample dividend.'[4]

Yet this survey was not observation in the usual clinical sense. Observation in medicine belonged to a certain structure of perception (the Panopticon) which analysed and described enclosed bodies. As Sheldon pointed out, medicine usually deals with the ill or possibly ill and therefore assumes these typical of the whole. But the community random sample revealed :'Those individuals who are ill and know they are ill, but have no intention of doing anything about it, as well as those who never have been ill.'[5]

Yet, interesting as the findings certainly were, it was the technique that held the greatest fascination for Sheldon. The random sample survey made accessible and intelligible to the medical gaze that which had remained hidden. 'Perhaps one of the deepest impressions left in my mind after conducting the survey is the fundamental importance of the random sample.'[6]

Other surveys followed that of Sheldon. In 1955 Hobson & Pemberton, in *The health of the elderly at home*, reported a similar survey of the health of old people.[7] Thompson, Low & McKeown reported a health survey of old people in Birmingham, in 1951.[8] Ferguson studied 300 old people receiving domiciliary care in Glasgow.[9] Prompted by the appearance of the health problems of old age in the field of medical visibility, many regional health boards established geriatric advisory committees, some of which, in an attempt to identify the extent of the problem of illness in old age, conducted their own surveys. Sheffield Regional Health Board, for example, carried out a survey in 1950 and published it in 1951.[10] 'So much knowledge of old age, not only in its medical field but also in its social field, has to be obtained through surveys', Sheldon pointed out to the 3rd Congress of the International Association of Gerontology held in London in 1954. 'A survey is really an aspect of the study of natural history'.[11]

A temporal gaze

When Sheldon claimed that the survey was an aspect of natural history he under-estimated the nature and power of the survey. The survey was not simply a mechanical technique, but a technology through which power operated as a positive force: the survey created a discourse, a practice, a reality. In this sense, the survey was not just an aspect of 'natural history' but a means of constituting and sustaining the very conception of 'natural history' as applied to illness.

In traditional clinical medicine, the natural history of an illness was assessed against the norm: when the illness was worsening, when it was improving, or when it had disappeared, could all be evaluated against the constancy of the norm. Within the temporal gaze of geriatrics, however, the norm was no longer absolute, no longer universal for all ages, but differed for those aged 7 months, 17 and 70 years. The norm was therefore replaced as a referrent by the normal. As Agate pointed out 'normal senescence' could only be identified by establishing whether changes in an old person were 'normal *for his years*'[12] (italics in original).

Post-war geriatrics thus stressed a temporal element in the clinical gaze. Geriatrics was not represented by a momentary frame as caught in the diagnosis, rather, it established an assessment and surveillance over time and space which had as its referrent an ever-changing criterion. In traditional clinical practice, diagnosis preceded treatment, but in geriatrics, as Howell observed, 'sometimes prognosis is more important than diagnosis'.[13] The doctor should ask: 'What is the future of this patient?'

(rather than what is the future of this disease). Disease in geriatrics was a sequence rather than a static entity: 'It is a moving film not merely a still photograph. What matters most is the direction in which the patient is going and the speed at which he is travelling. His exact position at any moment is less important.'[14]

The corollary of this perception of illness as a trajectory with constantly changing referrents was the model of care that geriatrics offered. Geriatrics differed from general medicine in that it had to 'continue supervision and management for a long period'.[15] For some geriatricians the specialty was not so much age- as morbidity-related.[16] Geriatrics discovered the chronic disease as a model for its practice and, in time, claims were made that it should be the specialty of disability and rehabilitation and therefore able to treat the young chronic sick too.[17]

It is important to separate the notion of chronicity from the morbidity group of chronic illness. 'Chronic' is no more than an adjective long used in medicine to describe a symptom, sign or illness which existed over a long time period, whereas chronic illness is a recent fabrication of a medical gaze which played on and between bodies. Thus, while it would be correct to claim that acute illness has been replaced by chronic disease as the principal problem of medical practice over the last three decades, it would be mistaken to ascribe this shift to technological advance and the elimination of acute infections, as has become fashionable. The problem is, as always, a political one: medical power has invented a new domain of illness which both derives from and justifies surveillance over time, yet medicine cannot be seen to have created its own object. An explanation of the change in morbidity spectrum has therefore been constructed from the elements of public knowledge that medicine has available. The notion of scientific progress establishes a history of an earlier age in which the major medical problems were acute and of their demise through a technical triumph whose cost, rather than creation, has been a new morbidity group. The medical gaze has established a domain of medical reality and with it the surveillance apparatus of support groups and social networks which act both to sustain and monitor the new temporally ordered medical space.[18]

Besides the constant surveillance demanded by chronic disease – with its acute exacerbations and temporary remissions – two other aspects of illness were used to justify geriatrics' monitoring gaze. First, as the survey had shown, many old people with illnesses chose, for various reasons, not to use medical services. This 'under-reporting' of illness, various geriatricians suggested, made screening of so-called 'normal' people particularly important.[19] Second, in old people, 'illness comes on insidiously with less clamant symptoms than in the young and in an individual who may well already have many minor ailments'.[20] These various factors – the ever-changing referrent, the clinical iceberg and the nature of geriatric illness – taken together, indicated the importance of a comprehensive basis for the organisation of geriatric services. As Anderson pointed out, geriatric medicine was clinical, social, preventive and remedial. 'Individuals discovered in the community must be supervised for life.'[21]

Unknown illnesses would have to be ascertained, preventive measures deployed to identify quickly the nascent signs of illness and to encourage health. 'Prevention of illness is the most important aspect of future work in the management of elderly people and the methodology of preventive geriatrics is based on the belief that the self-reporting of illness is not a satisfactory method of detecting illness at an early stage.'[22] Supervision would need to be carried out by a wide-ranging health care team. Hospitals, out-patient facilities and community services would need to be closely integrated to keep a watchful eye over the community of the elderly at risk; Andrews and his colleagues argued that this integration could best be achieved around the health centre, particularly if the 38% of old people they had identified as having unmet needs were to be provided for.[23]

The geriatric gaze over the domestic, as well as the hospitalised lives of the elderly, was in part through necessity in that so much chronic disease existed in the community. However, the geriatrician's concern with the elderly at home also arose because it was the domestic situation on which was articulated both the various techniques of long-term surveillance and the decipherment of the illnesses themselves. Foucault has shown, in *The birth of the clinic*, the close parallels with the localisation of the illness and its preferred place of treatment.[24] In the early eighteenth century the hospital was held to be a place where the nature and manifestations of disease were distorted: 'no hospital disease is a pure disease . . . the natural locus of disease is the natural locus of life – the family'.[25] On the other hand, at the end of the eighteenth century, when disease had been respatialised from its general and diverse manifestations in the body to specifically localisable tissue pathology, there was a concurrent shift in the point of observation from the home to the neutral domain of the hospital.

In post-war geriatrics, pathology was not so much localised, as in an open field of perception: illness, as the survey revealed, had an ever-changing distribution and relationship to the biography and social relationships of the patient. A hospitalised patient could not demonstrate how the disease would affect ordinary function nor how the various coping mechanisms which the patient might draw upon could actually work on discharge. Surely, Agate argued, 'the best place for elderly people is at home?'[26]

The organisational pattern of geriatrics, therefore, reflected the tension between its origins and principal workload in the hospital and the discourse which stressed the importance of the home. The day hospital was a device which enabled both surveillance from a hospital base and the maintenance of old people in their own homes.[27] Geriatricians encouraged domiciliary visiting, 'five-day wards' and tended to oppose long stays in hospitals or, where these were inevitable, to recreate certain features of the domestic ambience on the hospital ward. It was only in such a setting that the illness could be correctly observed in its natural context: a slight weakness in hospital could manifest itself as a functional impairment at home, an affective disorder might even be a result of the 'distorting' hospital environment.[28]

Moreover, the importance assigned the psycho–social context of illness, its expression and the various modes of coping which it necessitated, ensured that the geriatric gaze was also exercised over the social environment. 'Geriatric medicine is more closely involved with the social circumstances of its patients than is the medicine and surgery of those in the more active productive age groups. There is hardly a geriatric case in which the patient's mode of living can be discounted.'[29] The geriatric 'method' required, first, that a patient shall be considered as 'an important individual with a community identity';[30] the 'much more recent' idea that was employed in geriatrics was that 'every individual must be considered in relation to his environment'.[31]

The norm and the normal

The survey was the mechanism by which the essential problematic of geriatrics was discovered. The survey revealed the distribution of illness in the community; it enabled need to be identified; it assessed the social context of illness; it guided the deployment of services. Yet perhaps its major impact was on the conceptualisation of the normal. Hobson & Pemberton, in their survey published in 1955, for example, reported that the relationship between hypertension and symptoms was not as had been assumed by clinicians; the community survey of morbidity revealed that hypertension could be present without symptoms and symptoms could be present without hypertension. They also reported a wider range of 'normal' biochemistry than was usually supposed.[32]

This wide range of 'normal biochemical values' in the elderly obviously posed difficulties in interpretation. The problem, in a nutshell, as Jordan pointed out in 1956, was the difficulty of finding any old person without some biochemical abnormalities.[33] Consequently, he argued, 'subjects tend to be chosen as "normal" in respect of a particular investigation because they suffer from no conditions known to cause that particular investigation to yield abnormal results'. Yet, as Jordan was also aware, this procedure presented a logical difficulty in that it 'supposes a previous knowledge of the normal values for the particular investigation under consideration'.[34] In other words, it was a circular argument: normal biochemical values would be found in normal people who in turn would be defined as having normal biochemical values.

The survey reconstructed the normal. The survey analysed and described the characteristics of the social body of old people and, in so doing, dispensed with the dichotomy of the normal and the abnormal. Instead, it discovered that old people could be assigned to a point in a conceptual space characterised by a 'continuous distribution curve' of health.[35]

In mapping this conceptual space, geriatrics closely resembled paediatrics and indeed paediatrics provided a useful mode. Geriatrics, it was thought, could be 'defined in much the same way as paediatrics'[36] and in as much as it was 'a comparable subject and if it is to be developed both in respect of research and practice, it will require similar specialised cultivation'.[37] Geriatrics would be a separate discipline from general medicine 'just as paediatrics developed from the demonstration by Ashby, Still & Thompson that clinical efforts were frustrated without understanding biological modification by age'.[38] Where growth and development had provided the crucial cognitive and clinical dimension for paediatrics, so gerontology, the science of the study of ageing, could underpin the new geriatrics.[39]

Yet gerontology was only one part of geriatrics: the other was clinical experience as drawn from medicine in general;[40] and where gerontology, in its surveys, discovered the considerable range of normal variation in the ageing trajectory, clinical medicine attempted to evaluate that same trajectory by reference to the norm. Geriatrics, therefore, perhaps more than any of the other disciplines of the survey, created a discourse which juxtaposed the norm to the normal.

It was clear to Exton-Smith, in his textbook of 1955, that the norm by which the pathological was to be identified would arise from a 'knowledge of the physiological (i.e., normal) variation corresponding to the structural atrophy of organs and tissues'.[41] This particular knowledge, however, was difficult to establish in that 'such variation may pass into abnormality of function by hardly perceptible gradation'. Moreover, variations in involution could at times be so accentuated as to 'become pathological and result in a state which is obviously a departure from old age'.[42]

In his textbook of 1963, Agate similarly stressed the importance of the normal: 'the first step towards dealing rationally with elderly people is to have a clear conception of what ought to be accepted as normal'.[43] But this was not easy for 'morbidity increases with age and the physiological shades almost imperceptibly into the pathological'. The term 'senility', he suggested, should not be used as it did not distinguish between pathological processes and the characteristics of physiological ageing.

Isaacs, in 1965, argued that 'the main concern of the geriatrician is to decide whether a change which he detects in an old person is "normal" or "abnormal"' – though this distinction could not easily be made.[44] Tunbridge, in 1966, confirmed that there was 'an urgent need to establish true normals'.[45] Anderson felt that these 'true normals' could be established by dividing different ageing trajectories into normal and abnormal ageing. Though he acknowledged 'that "normal" attributes change with age',[46] he still believed that there existed in old age 'a super class of people who represent normal ageing almost untouched by disease'.[47] Yet how was this ageing elite to be identified? For Anderson, normal ageing would be characterised by the 'average values and scatter for all anatomical, physiological and biochemical attributes . . . for as near healthy individuals as we can obtain'.[48] Healthy individuals would define normal ageing while normal ageing would indicate healthy individuals. Understandably, Anderson concluded that 'the search for "normality" is still continuing'.[49]

By the late 1970s, however, this view was under attack. Coni and his co-authors, in 1977, pointed out that the notion of a 'biological elite' was misleading in that it represented but one extreme of a continuous distribution curve of health.[50] Also in 1977, Adams acknowledged that 'differentiation of "normal" from "pathological" ageing is often artificial but it is useful to distinguish preventable or reversible disease from age changes which are irreversible and have to be accepted, and it helps to simplify consideration of the ageing process to think of it in this way'.[51]

In 1948, when he carried out his survey of old people, Sheldon assessed social factors by questionnaire and was 'entirely subjective' in his evaluation of their physical state. He graded his respondents, normal, normal-plus or abnormal, in relation to their age. The use of this 'subjective' technique was justified on methodological grounds – a fuller, more 'objective' assessment would have been more difficult, expensive and time consuming.[52] Indeed Amulree, some years earlier, had identified the difficulty when he noted that: 'When people grow old there is a very narrow borderline between sickness and health.'[53]

Yet what in the immediate post-war years had appeared as an intransigent methodological problem, had, some 30 years later, been reformulated as a problem of clinical strategy. The assumptions of clinical medicine, such that there was a clear differentiation between health and disease, that diseases existed as separate entities, that disease could be recognised by clinical and laboratory study, or that precise diagnosis preceded treatment, were not necessarily true for geriatrics. As Isaacs argued in 1978: 'the ability to define the "normal" becomes neither a matter of semantics nor statistics, but a burning issue to be decided afresh at every clinical intervention'.[54]

10

A community gaze

The main manifestations of the extended disciplinary apparatus in the post-war medical world were in certain disciplines which, because of their proximity to the tactics of the survey, were invested with a new approach to illness, patients and health care delivery; those parts of medicine – particularly hospital based – which were components of a panoptic vision, also started to be transformed by the new procedures of the survey. The Goodenough Report of 1944 had recommended the establishment of departments of social medicine within medical schools[1] and it was from within these departments that a revitalised epidemiology was to emerge and shape a medical perception of the social.

In 1957 Morris published the first edition of his *Uses of epidemiology*.[2] In contrast to clinical medicine, he argued, the unit of study of epidemiology was the population or group not the individual. Yet, although epidemiology had the group as its object, it was primarily a method, a way of analysing and perceiving medical reality. Morris claimed it was a perception which asked different questions and obtained different answers from those asked by clinicians. Sometimes, the epidemiologist 'asks questions which the clinician also asks, and gets different information in reply. Often the epidemiologists can ask questions that cannot be asked in clinical medicine at all.'[3]

Morris suggested that epidemiology had seven separate, though related, uses in medicine. It could provide historical evidence for changes in diseases and their distributions, enable the diagnosis of the health of the community, aid the study of the working of the health service, help calculate the risks for individuals of various diseases, complete the clinical picture and natural history of diseases, help identify new syndromes and search for the causes of disease. The survey, particularly of non-infective disease, provided the basis of all these various uses.

The chief growth point in epidemiology, Morris suggested, was in surveys of morbidity: 'the study of morbidity is expanding rapidly and it is becoming a main interest of Public Health since mortality is progressively less useful in the diagnosis of public health'.[4] Morris himself, in his first published work in 1941, had reported a health survey of a Midlands factory workforce.[5] The Medical Research Council had surveyed the haemoglobin of 16 000 people in 1943.[6] Magee & Milligan, in 1951, reported the haemoglobin levels of 2087 'unselected' women attending welfare clinics and, from the data, constructed ante-natal and post-natal haemoglobin 'curves'[7]. A year later Berry & Magee published haemoglobin levels of a school population, of housewives 'randomly' selected in the street, and of a random sample of workers earning less than £1000 per annum.[8]

The interim results of a more ambitious project, the ascertainment of all pulmonary tuberculosis in the Rhondda Valley, were published by Cochrane and his co-workers in 1952.[9] 89% of the population were reported to have been x-rayed. Higgins and his co-workers, in 1956, reported a comparative random survey of 245 men for respiratory symptoms and pulmonary disability in an English industrial town (Leigh) to establish whether miners in the Welsh Rhondda had excess respiratory morbidity.[10] The College of General Practitioners, in one of the first of its 'collective investigations', with the help of the Ministry of Health, carried out a similar respiratory survey on an age-stratified random sample of patients drawn from practice lists.[11]

In 1952 Getting and his co-workers surveyed a diabetic clinic in Gloucester.[12] In 1953 Tunbridge reported a survey of patients attending the Leeds diabetic clinic.[13] Every fifth patient was asked to keep a daily diary of their diet which was, in turn, monitored by social-worker visits at the beginning, during and at the end of the survey. Redhead, in 1960, in a survey of 20% of his practice list, confirmed American reports of 'a reservoir of undiagnosed diabetes in the practice population'.[14] Walker & Kerridge reported similar results in a survey from Ibstock,[15] as did Harkness from Halstead[16] and the College of General Practitioners from Birmingham.[17] Butterfield & Keen carried out a large survey in a search for unrecognised diabetics in Bedford in 1961.[18]

Doll and his co-workers reported on the prevalence of peptic ulcer in different occupations in 1951;[19] Stewart & Hughes examined the prevalence of tuberculosis among shoe-makers, also in 1951;[20] Mial and his co-workers looked at the prevalence of rheumatoid arthritis in South Wales in the early 1950s;[21] Pickering and his co-workers reported on the distribution of blood pressure in a 'normal' population in 1954.[22]

This great interest in community morbidity, thought Morris, was but 'one illustration of the modern community's need to know itself, a need whose wide recognition – anew – represents a striking change in the climate of opinion.... The more complex a society, the more does it need an inquisitive intelligence service to diagnose itself.'[23] To this end, the survey represented the ideal technique and, moreover, Morris claimed, 'the renaissance of sociology . . . is opening up the possibility for public health of an altogether more penetrating social analysis'.[24]

For the clinician in hospital practice, these prevalence surveys provided 'accurate information as to the real numbers of diseased people in any population', thus setting their hospital work load in context. The surveys could also be used to obtain direct evidence concerning: 'The natural history of a disease, the true frequency of its various manifestations, or its association with other diseases, and they may throw light on the aetiology of a disease.'[25] As Witts, the Nuffield Professor of Medicine at Oxford, argued, one of the main functions of 'group research' was to broaden contact with sick people and to ensure that the clinical scientist's mind remained open to the major problems of human disease.[26]

The problem of the borderline case

The increasing post-war medical interest in morbidity (as against mortality), together with the results of various surveys, created problems of definition: the counting of deaths was relatively straightforward compared with measuring illness. In 1966, for example, in a report on the Bedford survey of diabetics, Keen pointed out that although 4% of the sample had glycosuria (sugar in the urine – a diagnostic test for diabetes) many of these 'diabetics' did not show an abnormal glucose tolerance curve (another diagnostic test for diabetes).[27] The question, as Keen noted, was: had the survey in using glycosuria as the diagnostic test uncovered 'true' diabetics; or was the abnormal tolerance curve – even in the absence of glycosuria – the mark of the diabetic? In short, the findings of the survey had led to a questioning of 'our concepts of diabetes as a disease entity'.[28]

In 1924 Faber had published a book entitled *Nosography in internal medicine*, in which he carefully documented the historical rise and triumph of a particular medical perception which accepted an ontological conception of disease.[29] In classifying various morbid events into disease categories, the physician believed he was identifying discrete entities existing independently of other life forms. Crookshank, an early exponent of the new social medicine (and of the value of psychotherapy), had challenged this assumption in 1939, arguing that diseases were but quantitative deviations from the normal.[30] Nevertheless, at least until the post-war period, medical opinion held firmly to the belief that diseases or pathology were qualitatively different from the normal or physiological processes which enabled the organism to sustain life.

By the early 1950s, however, various American writers had virtually dismissed the ontological view: King, for example, argued that 'disease is an arbitrary designation'[31], and Riese boldly claimed that 'everyone agrees that the nosological entity or any other schema is an abstraction'.[32] In England, Ryle challenged the traditional view of the normal, in 1947, with illustrations of 'normal variability' drawn from various surveys.[33] 'Health and disease know no sharp boundary', he claimed, 'variability, both in time and in the species, is one of the most distinctive and necessary attributes of life, which thus admits no constant and no norm.'[34] Yet, in 1955, Cohen could point out that 'the concept of disease as a "clinical entity" still dominates much of our textbook descriptions' and that minds were 'still shackled with the concept of disease as "entities"'.[35] The prolonged and often acrimonious debate about the nature of essential hypertension, during subsequent years, was a powerful illustration of the prejudice Cohen had identified.

In 1954 Pickering and his co-workers published a paper on arterial blood pressure in the general population.[36] Over the next decade, the findings achieved considerable notoriety and led to a barrage of argument and insult between some of the leading physicians of the day, such that Pickering could with some justification claim in the *Lancet* that, 'nowadays odium scholasticum is usually discreetly veiled but your readers are being treated to a splendid display'.[37]

Pickering recorded the blood pressures of all patients attending clinics for varicose veins, diseases of the skin, fractures, orthopaedics diseases and dental treatment at St Mary's Hospital during six months of 1951. He found that blood pressure in these patients (who, he claimed, were representative of the general population) showed a normal distribution rising with age. Moreover, because there was no sharp demarcation between blood pressures which had traditionally been accepted as normal and those thought of as being pathological (essential hypertension), Pickering and his co-workers were 'led to doubt whether there is any justification other than that of convenience, for drawing a line dividing normal from abnormal pressure. It would seem in fact, that the term essential hypertension represents no more than that section of the population in which the arterial pressure exceeds an arbitrary value and in which no other disease is found to account for the arterial pressures observed. According to where we draw the line, so we can make essential hypertension as common or as rare as we wish.'[38]

The survey, in mapping the characteristics of a total population, had uncovered the continuity of its physiological parameters. If so-called disease states were continuous with general population measurements, then how could disease be a separate, discrete entity? 'This conception of the nature of essential hypertension', Pickering noted, 'appears to be a novel one, though it is so obvious that it is difficult to understand why it has not been clearly stated before.'[39] Against the older notion of separate populations of healthy and ill, Pickering presented the concept of continuous distribution of measurable traits in total populations, and the concept of normal variability to cope with quantitative differences.

A distinct boundary between physiology and pathology belonged to the perceptual gaze of the Panopticon which sought to enclose and monitor deviants; in the new idea of continuous distributions, the normal became problematic and illness was reduced to the 'semi-philosophical notion of a physiological abnormality' as McMichael dismissively suggested.[40] It was precisely this encounter, between a clinical gaze which dichotomised and the tactics of the survey which uncovered continuity, that focused attention on the borderline between normality and abnormality. If the discourse which characterised general practice in the post-war world was on trivia and that which characterised geriatrics was on chronic illness, then in general medicine it was the discourse on the borderline case.

As well as undermining the ontological status of the concept of disease, the borderline case became an accepted category in community prevalence studies. It was a classification which, in practical terms, made the problematic boundary between normality and pathology manageable (the Bedford survey of diabetes classified all blood sugar estimations of 120–200 MG % as borderline cases)[41] and at the same time caused the researchers to try and sharpen their definitions and research instruments to minimise the size of this basically unsatisfactory category.

Screening for disease, which had developed in rudimentary form in the early twentieth-century manifestations of the Dispensary (such as the school health service inspection clinic), came into more general use with the post-war discovery through the survey of the vast extent of community morbidity. Multi-phasic screening was carried out in the United States in the early 1950s[42] and reported in Britain in the 1960s.[43] In 1968 the Nuffield Foundation published a volume on the value of screening for different diseases[44] and in the same year Butterfield, in his Rock Carling Lecture on priorities in medicine, advocated a new emphasis on screening in health care delivery.[45] Moreover, he discussed the problem of screening for a continuously distributed variable, only one extreme of which constituted disease, in terms of controls and borderlines.

Morris, in the second edition of *Uses of epidemiology* published in 1964, expanded his section on screening to explore the category of the subclinical. He stressed the importance of penetrating to the 'early minor stages' and then further back to the precursors of disease and to its predispositions. Such devices served to further refine certain elements of an ambiguous borderline which, under certain conditions might remain essentially normal and under others might translate themselves into full-blown disease states.[46] The ambiguity was thereafter couched in a new terminology of screening which identified true positives and false positives, true negatives and false negatives.

Multiple causes

One of the seven uses of epidemiology that Morris identified was the search for the causes of diseases. In this section he laid particular emphasis on the notion of multiple causes rather than on the idea that individual diseases had single causes – a belief, Morris suggested, which arose from germ theory in the nineteenth century. The notion of multiple causes was, moreover, a new discovery: 'the notion of "pattern of causes" is a relatively modern statement'.[47]

In 1942, in a paper entitled 'Aetiology: a plea for wider concepts and new study', Ryle argued that while Pasteur and other pioneers in bacteriology had been of immense benefit to medicine they had 'a peculiarly limiting effect upon the vision and the practice of many medical men'.[48] Specifically, they had 'compelled a neglect of the associated causal factors without which no disease can have its being. They also fostered a belief in or search for single determining causes where none exist.'[49]

Until the inter-war years the concept of cause or aetiology was dominated by a search for and belief in a single cause. Models of causality in medical discourse, such as in Muir's *Textbook of pathology* (3rd edition, 1933), relied on bacteria and viruses: 'we speak of the tubercle bacillus as the cause of tuberculosis in the sense that the introduction of the bacillus is ordinarily followed by the disease and that the latter is not met with apart from the bacillus'.[50] However, it was also becoming apparent in the inter-war years that the notion of a single cause required some qualification: a medicine with an extended gaze – especially to the mind and to the community – uncovered other factors apparently causally implicated. Muir's textbook, in 1933, accepted the need to acknowledge these factors, though it did so in terms which did not fundamentally challenge the dominance of single cause theory: 'with regard to many conditions we have to speak of predisposing, contributing and auxiliary causes'.[51]

By the sixth edition of Muir's textbook, in 1951, the position had significantly changed. It was claimed that, with the exception of 'certain infectious diseases, it is no longer supposed that each disease or illness has a single specific cause which is the *sine qua non* of the state'.[52] This point had been made earlier, in the fifth edition of 1941, as far as the aetiology of tumours was concerned. The cause of tumours, in the 1933 edition, was held to be largely unknown though 'chronic irritability' was suggested as a possibility. By 1941, however, a multi-factorial aetiology was clearly stated:

'one often hears the phrase "the cause of cancer" but so far as the starting of the growth is concerned there is no one cause; there are many causes'.[53]

Many infectious diseases were acknowledged as having 'multiple causes' only, by the 1951 edition. For tuberculosis, the claim that the tubercle bacillus was always present was tempered by the observation that 'the converse is not necessarily true and the presence of the bacillus is not invariably followed by the disease'.[54] By implication, at least, the disease had more than the bacillus as its cause. Perhaps the argument was put more clearly in the general discussion of the cause of pathology (in the 1951 edition) which, while still using the germ-theory model, acknowledged that 'if bacteria are to be regarded as the *seeds* of disease, it is now realised clearly that the *soil* is also fundamentally important'.[55]

Although it took so long to reach the pathological textbooks, the discovery of the 'soil' in which the tubercle seed could take root had occurred earlier in the century. The Dispensary vision had discovered the 'soil' of disease when it turned its gaze to the social milieu. A perception which measured and analysed social relationships and social environments was also a perception which inevitably invented a multi-factorial aetiology of disease. It was epidemiologists such as Morris who pressed it on the profession; the new specialists in social medicine, such as Ryle, who argued its value; and the techniques of the survey, such as the randomised control trial, which in the very notion of randomised controls acknowledge the causal influence of the extraneous variable.

For Ryle, in 1942, the concept of 'multiple factors' was especially useful in understanding chronic illness because in these diseases, factors such as 'age, sex, habits and occupation' were part of a 'temporal' dimension which continually sustained and affected the long-term course of the illness.[56] Multiple causes were less important in acute diseases as their 'quick tempo' allowed so little time for these other factors to have an effect.

The notion of causality belongs, Durkheim would have us believe, with space and time as the basic categories of human thought which have their origin in the social milieu.[57] Just as the distribution of the social group defined space and the ritual of its ceremonies delineated time, so the experience of external events established causality. When the group was paramount and individual identity non-existent, causality could only be seen in fatalistic terms; with increasing individualisation through the division of labour causality became contingent. Thus a more sophisticated separation of individual identities and a more complex interactional model can be read into the invention of multi-causal explanations. Identity was not given simply by physical separation but also in psychological relationships through which the effect of one individual on another was both contingent and reciprocal. Multi-factorial aetiology was an invention of a social gaze. 'Much that is truly aetiology' Ryle concluded 'extends beyond the relatively confined province of pathology and invades the broader territory of social science.'[58] Or, as MacKay noted in 1951, if 'the search for specific (aetiological) agents halted the progress of social medicine then the role of nutrition, psychological medicine, stress and other trends reawakened interest in "broader domains of aetiology"'.[59]

Illness, in the post-war years, began to be temporally and spatially distributed, not in a physical domain, but in a community. The community was the term deployed to describe that truly social space that had emerged in the calculated gap between bodies: a network of interrelated and interdependent points between which power was exercised reflexively. Comprehensive health care in Britain, from 1948, and the contemporary invention and importance placed on community care are simply manifestations of a new diagram of power which spreads its pervasive gaze throughout a society.

11

Subjective bodies

The deployment of the new technology of the survey in the post-war medical world resulted in the crystallisation of new patterns of medical specialisation. Whereas, previously, medical specialisation had been structured around the examination, description and analysis of the body of the patient, the new specialties were deployed in the spaces between people. In paediatrics the clinical gaze was deployed around the body of the normal child; in psychiatry it was mainly deployed around the coping strategies of ordinary people; in general practice the gaze turned from the grossly pathological to the minor and transient changes in health perception which hardly left their mark on the body of the patient; in geriatrics the gaze was deployed over time, in the observation of chronic illness and of the longitudinal bodily changes which required constant monitoring and interpretation.

Together, these new specialties created a constant web of observation around the normal individual and, in so doing, at times coalesced to create yet more specialties. In 1965, McKeown, in advocating some degree of specialisation in general practice, suggested four areas in which GPs should practice: adults, children, the elderly and obstetric cases.[1] The idea of a GP paediatrician and a GP geriatrician were points at which the new disciplines of the survey intersected. The GP obstetrician, moreover, was another amalgamation of two surveillance technologies in that the obstetric component provided, in its ante-natal care, a constant gaze over a normal (yet essentially problematic) pregnancy. In the Court Report, of 1976, paediatrics again extended its reach in recommending specialist GP paediatricians and a special community role for paediatrics.[2] In the same way, geriatrics in recent decades has reached out beyond the hospital to an increasing community and domiciliary role.

There were important links between psychiatry and general practice, especially in the analysis and identification of the neuroses. For many GPs the bulk of their time is spent practising 'community psychiatry' whilst psychiatrists show increasing interest in community morbidity and in holding out-patient clinics in general practice.[3] Out of psychiatry and paediatrics has come a separate specialty, child psychiatry[4] and despite its relative low status psychogeriatrics is an established and growing discipline.[5]

If the panoptic vision created individual bodies by objectifying them through their analysis and description, then the dense web of surveillance around and between bodies, as shown by the constant gaze of the new disciplines of the survey and the renewed interest of clinical medicine in the borderline case, created a mechanism for constituting bodies in a different fashion. The new body is not a disciplined object constituted by a medical gaze which traverses it, but a body fabricated by a gaze which surrounds it: the new body is one held in constant juxtaposition to other bodies, a body constituted by its social relationships and relative mental functioning, a body, of necessity, of a subject rather than an object.

The doctor–patient relationship

In 1944 the Goodenough Committee produced a report on medical education in which the patient was hardly mentioned.[6] To be sure, the medical student had to be taught how to diagnose disease in his patients, but the patient was viewed essentially as a passive object in which was contained interesting pathology. Thus, in the introductory clinical course in which clinical skills were to be mastered, the Goodenough Committee emphasised accuracy in recognising the physical signs of disease: 'general pathological states should be shown and their signs and symptoms identified on the living patient'[7] (in contradistinction to the dead patient of the post-mortem room). It was felt that training in 'the taking of a complete history of a patient's illness' should take place in undergraduate medical education but no further guidance was offered nor any indication given that this procedure was at all problematic. Indeed, the form of the interaction envisaged between doctor and patient was perhaps illustrated by the comment that at the beginning of the course students rarely know how to 'interrogate' a patient.[8]

Some twenty years later, in the *Report on the Royal Commission of Medical Education* (Todd Report), the term 'taking the history' was self-consciously placed in inverted commas.[9] It was pointed out that 'there is a great deal more to this than simply asking a series of prescribed questions and checking the accuracy of the answers. Students must be aware of the factors which impede or distort communication, factors such as limitations of vocabulary, cultural attitudes and social prejudices.'[10] Between the Goodenough Report and the Todd Report, the patient can be seen as entering a new relationship with the doctor – a relationship which might be rewarding, important, difficult or therapeutic, but one which some twenty years earlier had been ignored.

It is in this new discourse around the discovery of an inherently problematic relationship, after World War II, that there can be discerned the lines of a reconstructed doctor–patient interaction and the fabrication of the patient as a subject. Two lines of analysis of the doctor–patient relationship can be identified: the first concerns the mapping of the social space between doctor and patient, the second, the crystallisation and localisation of the 'problem' within that space.

Communication across a social space

From its foundation, in 1925, the *British Journal of Venereal Diseases* was dominated by papers on the clinical and pathological aspects of venereology. The total lack of mention of the patient in the early years as other than the carrier of pathology, reflected the irrelevance of the patient's individuality for the practice of venereology. In 1932, however, the patient received separate mention for the first time. Frazer, in a paper entitled 'The problem of the defaulter', analysed 50 replies to a questionnaire he had sent to a group of defaulters from VD treatment.[11] He concluded from his study that it was important to 'impress on all patients at *intervals* the necessity of treatment' and that the patient should 'repeat all directions so no misunderstanding can occur'.[12]

In Foucault's analysis of the emergence, towards the end of the eighteenth century, of the body as an object which could be used, transformed and rendered docile, part of the mechanism by which passivity was achieved was the newly discovered clinical examination.[13] In that the clinical examination involved an invasion of 'private' body space, in that it involved an analysis and dissection of the body and in that it subjected the whole body – its surface, its crevices, its insides, its workings – to a medical gaze, then the body (and hence the patient) was constituted as a discrete, though passive, object. The clinical examination thus fabricated the body and through its rituals privatised it and made it passive. If the patient accepted this gaze then its effects were achieved yet even resistance to the gaze produced the same result because resistance was itself based on the notion of the body as a discrete and personalised object. Thus the body was held in, and constituted by, a field of surveillance from which it could not escape.

In Frazer's paper on defaulters, however, the body is analysed in terms other than passivity. In addition to being the docile carrier of disease, the patient achieves a tentative identity as a potential defaulter. The patient is not simply an object which will conform; it possesses, in its potential for default, a germ of idiosyncracy. Hence derived the need, as expressed in Frazer's concluding advice on how to manage this danger, to begin to treat the patient as other than a wholly passive body, albeit one which, with the correct instructions, could be made passive.

In 1935, in the same journal, a series of four papers on default were published. Hanschell reported on 'The defaulting seaman',[14] Nichol on 'The defaulting prostitute'[15] and 'The defaulting travelling man',[16] and Nabarro on 'The defaulting child'.[17] In 1947 MacFarlane & Johns reported 'a medico–social analysis of 381 women patients' in an attempt to locate venereal disease defaulters from a social point of view.[18]

The perception of the patient as an actual or potential defaulter, represented a constant theme in post-war literature on the doctor–patient relationship. Yet within this continuing concern with default can be discerned the subtle changes through which the patient was being reconstituted. First, the negative, pejorative 'defaulter' was reanalysed in a much more complex and subtle discourse on 'compliance' suggesting that obedience to medical advice could not be so starkly assumed. The patient was thereby transformed from someone who simply failed to follow advice to someone who chose whether or not to follow that advice. In this latter formulation, the element of choice stands in contrast to the docility of the patient as conceived in traditional medical discourse.

In an overview of patient non-compliance, in 1976, Ley examined four theories.[19] First, there was the 'personality hypothesis' which argued that non-compliance was a function of personality, attitude or demographic characteristics. Ley pointed out, however, that evidence in support of this hypothesis was weak; in addition, even if such links were to be 'incontrovertibly established, knowledge of them is of little practical use'.[20] The remaining three theories he claimed were more useful. The psychodynamic hypothesis posited that non-compliance would result if the 'deep' problem was not tackled; the interaction hypothesis placed the problem within the process in which doctor and patient negotiated the interview; the cognitive hypothesis (which Ley supported) presented the problem as one of memory and/or understanding.

In all these theories, however, there was a common element: the central problem was cast as one of communication and it was assumed that patients' dissatisfaction and non-compliance were directly a result of communication difficulties. In the 1960s and 1970s, therefore, the older problems of default and compliance became points on which were articulated the new concerns with 'effective' communication.

The problem of communication can be traced back to the recognition of widespread anxiety among patients in the inter-war years.[21] By 1946 it was believed that anxiety could be combated with adequate reassurance by the doctor. Cole felt that 'many people today carry unnecessary burdens of anxiety about their health which limit their happiness and activity', simply because they had not been given adequate reassurance about their prognosis.[22] Armstrong, in pointing out the neglect of the management and handling of patients in the medical curriculum over the previous 50 years, argued for the importance of allaying patients' anxieties through reassurance.[23] Parkinson thought that patients were inclined towards a 'sombre prognosis', with consequent undue apprehension, anxiety and fear.[24]

By 1960, however, the task of reassuring patients had begun to be widened. Meares argued that 'the whole business of communication with the patient is something much more complex than our traditional concept of history-taking'.[25] He pointed to the importance of verbal, extra-verbal and non-verbal channels of communication between doctor and patient. In 1963 a Sub-Committee of the Central Health Services Council produced a pamphlet entitled *Communication between doctors, nurses and patients: an aspect of human relations in the hospital service*.[26] The Committee had been appointed in 1961 to improve information flow to the patient, although it concluded that little was known 'objectively' about patients and their reactions to treatment.[27] Yet, as the *Lancet* claimed, the patient needed 'someone he can call by name who will listen to his troubles, answer his questions and represent him in the medical world'.[28] A year later, in 1964, Cartwright, in a survey of hospital patients' attitudes to treatment, found that patients complained of lack of information more than anything else.[29]

In his discussion of communication with patients in the Rock Carling Lecture, 'Communication in medicine', Fletcher took compliance as his central theme.[30] He provided a brief discussion on 'acquiring information' but the bulk of the review was on 'giving information'. 'How can we improve our communication with patients?', Fletcher asked. 'The first thing is to recognise the problem. Few doctors realise how little of what they tell their patients may be understood or remembered.'[31]

Pathology and personality

The second strand in the new discourse on the doctor–patient relationship – and one which intertwined at various points with the problem of communication – was that of the shift in location of the medical problem and the invention of whole-person medicine. Brackenbury announced the 'new relationship arising out of the present outlook of medicine' in his book entitled *Patient and doctor*, published in 1935.[32] As Secretary of the British Medical Association through most of the inter-war period, Brackenbury had endorsed and espoused a wider 'social work' role for the GP such that he held it important that doctors should locate illness in its social context.[33] His view of the medical task was of a relationship between two personalities: 'the relationship between patient and doctor is not merely, between two persons, but between two personalities. . . . It is never the body which is out of health, but always the complete being.'[34]

Nevertheless, although Brackenbury advised a relationship of personalities based on whole-person medicine, the patient in his schema remains an object. In his discussion of 'what the patient expects', it is what the patient expects of the doctor, rather than what the patient expects of the relationship, which is discussed. The patient is construed as a passive object, expecting from the doctor certain qualities – knowledge, skill, carefulness, judgement, sympathy, understanding, moral character, and ethical conduct.[35] Moreover, the degree to which the 'new psychological outlook of medicine' was reflected in this new relationship was mainly to be found amongst general practitioners: the relationship between patient and specialist, as a product of the referral system, tended to be more 'indirect'.[36]

Brackenbury's perception of the patient as an object is further evidenced in his descriptions of what the doctor expects of the patient. Subjectivity, meaning, idiosyncracy, feelings, a social nexus – themes which were to dominate certain post-war analyses of the doctor–patient relationship – were absent. The doctor expected two responses from the patient, 'obedience and confidence – unless one may properly add as a third, the will to get better or the will to keep well'.[37]

Although Brackenbury's analysis of the doctor–patient relationship might seem somewhat mechanistic, it is representative of a new medical literature on the doctor–patient relationship which emerged in Britain during the 1930s at about the same time as the new medical psychology and its object, the neuroses, became increasingly salient. As the new discourse on mental instability, the ubiquity of the neuroses and the necessity for a general mental hygiene spread, so the patient, or at least some patients, became more than simple repositories of organic pathology. As Raven[38] and Campbell[39] pointed out, in 1932, the doctor must become aware of the patient's personality. The patient was not simply an object but a person, as Crichton-Miller put it, needing enlightenment and reassurance.[40]

In this reassessment of the patient's identity the psychoanalytic school had a role. Jones, one of the latter's leading members, observed in 1938 that 'there are few cases in which the unconscious mind of the patient does not play a part in the clinical situation'.[41] Yet perhaps more significant was the readiness with which other clinicians accepted the new psychology and its implications for the doctor–patient relationship. For example, Lett, the President of the Royal College of Surgeons, argued in 1939 that, in the past, students had had to rely on their natural gifts and instincts in their relationship with the patient. Now, with the advent of the new psychology the fundamentals of the relationship – sympathetic understanding, cheerfulness and confidence – would need more formal teaching.[42]

This is not to argue that during the 1930s the medical profession as a whole were persuaded of the new approach to the patient. Cassidy, for example, senior physician at St Thomas's thought the new analysis of the patient's personality a waste of time: 'what a lot of valuable time would be saved if our patients could be taught that all we want to hear from them is an account of their symptoms, as concise as possible and chronological!'[43] Yet even behind this apparent opposition lay a recognition of a new role for the patient. The patient could not give a clear history because the patient was no longer a passive body. The literature which recognised the value of an obscure history (because it told of the patient's personality), or the literature which opposed it (because it delayed finding the organic pathology), both belonged to the same discourse which, in its deployment, began to destroy the concept of the patient as a docile body.

If the pre-war discourse on the doctor–patient relationship established the bare outlines of a patient with a personality, then the post-war discourse, through the increasing respect it accorded that personality, began to further constitute the patient as subject. In 1948, for example, in the first paper of its kind in the *British Journal of Venereal Diseases*, Wittkower discussed the 'psychological aspects of venereal disease'.[44] He pointed out that he and Cowan, following similar American studies, had been asked by the War Office to investigate the personality, sex behaviour and 'driving forces' in a group of patients with venereal disease. He concluded by emphasising the importance of psycho–social considerations in understanding the problem. Wittkower also noted in his paper that he had written nothing about the patient's reaction to the diagnosis of venereal disease. This neglect was not because this problem was unimportant: in his study the patients had accepted the disease, he thought, 'philosophically'; but in civilians, the reaction was important as 'serious concern' was often expressed.[45] Some two years later, in 1950, in a review of 'some individual and social factors in venereal disease', Sutherland concluded that the social medicine approach must be applied to the study of venereal disease: 'the whole patient must be studied and treated as well as his infected tissues . . . every patient is anxious and disturbed'.[46]

Where the Goodenough Report on medical education, of 1944, had conceived of the patient entirely as an object, the Report of the Planning Committee of the Royal College of Physicians on medical education, in the same year, reflected some of these new concerns.[47] The Planning Committee stressed that the primary objective of the undergraduate course was to teach method: 'method for elucidating the facts concerning disease, method for welding these facts into an understanding of, and judgement on, the question at issue, method for testing the validity of this judgement'.[48] In this process the report acknowledged the importance of 'lecture-demonstrations and practical exercises in the method of history-taking and clinical examination', though detail was only provided on how the clinical examination should be taught.[49] Perhaps a clearer indication of the Committee's thinking was given in its discussion of the place of psychological medicine in the curriculum. Recognising that teaching in psychological matters was by and large defective, the Committee advocated that greater attention should be placed on 'an acute appreciation of human nature'; in particular it was felt essential that 'from the beginning of his clinical career, the student should be encouraged to study his patient's personality . . . just as he studies his patient's physical signs and the data on the temperature chart'.[50]

Thus, by the end of the 1940s, the medical gaze began to fix with more tenacity on the patient's personality. In 1949, Spence, the paediatrician, could argue that the 'doctor needs to know the individual ... he must understand him in many of [his] variations from the norm',[51] while in the same year Cairns, Professor of Surgery at Oxford, could reiterate that the good doctor 'studies the patient's personality as well as his disease'.[52]

By the mid 1950s the patient's personality had become sufficiently fixed in the medical field of visibility that some of its implications could be analysed. In 1955 Balint published a classic paper on 'The doctor, his patient and the illness'[53] (later expanded into a book of the same title[54]), in which he outlined some implications of the patient-as-subject for understanding patient behaviour and reactions to the doctor. In the same year, Järvinen, in a paper entitled 'Can ward rounds be a danger to patients with myocardial infarction?', argued that a higher mortality rate after a ward round might be caused by the patient's reaction to the psychological strain;[55] Ellison tacitly acknowledged the existence of the patient in a social network when he presented arguments in the *Lancet* for the importance of managing the coping problems of the patient's relatives;[56] and Clark-Kennedy, in pointing out the active part the patient must play in keeping healthy, effectively denounced the perception of the patient as a passive object.[57]

Whereas earlier the diagnostic function of medicine had created categories of patients with different diseases, the new medical gaze, which created a web of observation and concern around the idiosyncratic patient, established an individual identity. This is illustrated in venereology where Rogerson, for example, in 1951, identified venereophobia in certain patients: 'to the sufferer it is often more distressing than a real attack of gonorrhoea or syphilis to the average patient'.[58] In 1952 the Venerologist

Group Committee of the BMA, following a questionnaire sent to all venereologists, pronounced on the importance of social workers being an integral part of the venereal disease service.[59] In 1953, Horne, in an analysis of the 'contemporary defaulter', offered a more complex view of the problem than his predecessors some years earlier. 'The behaviour of persons under treatment and observation ... should be considered in planning the management of such patients.'[60] Thus gradually, the patient with venereal disease was reconstrued: from being simply a member of a particular group, he became an individual with unique characteristics. To be sure, venereal disease was still found to excess in the promiscuous, but it was now recognised that 'the promiscuous spring from every class of society and every type of home'.[61] Some people resisted the pressures on them, others did not, 'the individual character and psychological make-up being the determining factor. Each girl travels her personal byway to promiscuity.'[62]

In 1966, in a series of articles in *The Practitioner*, under the general heading of 'The doctor–patient relationship', Browne & Freeling offered a formalised analysis of the interaction between doctor and patient.[63] The articles were republished as a book in 1967 and a second edition was published in 1976.[64] In their writing, Browne & Freeling endorsed 'whole problem care' as the task of medicine, with the GP's role specifically 'to understand the whole of his patient's communication so that he could assess the whole person and be able to consider the effect of any intervention in an illness upon the whole life of his patient'.[65]

This approach was later endorsed by the teaching manual published by the Royal College of General Practitioners, in 1972, entitled *The future general practitioner*, in which the consultation became the axis on which all of general practice was based.[66] In the same year, a volume of papers from the First International Conference of the Balint Society, under the title *Patient-centred medicine*, further defined and celebrated the new importance of the patient within the practice of medicine.[67]

No better illustration of the enormity of the change that had come over medicine since the beginning of the century can be given than the changes in the manuals used for teaching clinical method. Perhaps the most famous of these is Hutchison's *Clinical methods*, first published in 1897.[68] The sixth edition, of 1916, had a brief section on 'the interrogation of the patient' in the chapter on 'case taking'. There the student was advised to be patient, allow the patient to tell their own stories (better to reach a correct diagnosis), not to ask leading questions (except to trap malingerers) and not to ask the same question twice. The twelfth edition, of 1949, was very much the same.[69] The sixteenth edition, of 1975, however, stressed the importance of the patient's social circumstances and commended Balint 'sensitivity groups' as a means of improving the doctor–patient relationship.[70] History-taking was not an interrogation but an art and above all 'a two-way business'. The importance of non-verbal communication was discussed; the fact that the doctor's touch may be seen as an attack or a caress was pointed out, and it was stressed that being a patient was an ordeal: evasiveness, it was argued, might be an expression of anxiety, or a presenting complaint merely a 'ticket' to gain entry to the relationship.[71]

Identity of the patient

In his discussion of the emergence of the 'individual' at the end of the eighteenth century, Foucault points out that the new (clinical) examination assured 'the great disciplinary functions of distribution and classification, maximum extraction of forces and time, continuous genetic accumulation, optimum combination of aptitudes and thereby the fabrication of cellular, organic, genetic and combinatory individuality'. In effect, the examination was 'at the centre of procedures that constitute the individual as effect and object of power, as effect and object of knowledge'.[72]

In similar fashion, the discourse on the doctor–patient relationship over the last few decades has, like the clinical examination, had an object and an effect. The clinical examination was a device for ordering bodies, which, in doing so, constituted them; the medical interview and relationship has become a comparable mechanism for analysing, and thereby fabricating, idiosyncratic patients. The medical discourse on default, compliance, personality, sensitivity, meanings, subjectivity, etc., has not simply been a device with which to explore certain problematic elements in the doctor–patient relationship: rather, the creation of the discourse has had the effect of constituting the very problems which it nominally set out to explore. A discourse on default constituted the patient as a potential defaulter; a discourse on communication rendered meanings between doctor and patient problematic; a discourse on personality established the centrality of patient subjectivity to the medical enterprise; and so on. In other words, in scrutinising the consequences and implications of accepting the patient-as-person, the discourse has fabricated that same patient. This 'whole person' is, therefore, the product of a series of smaller discourses (on compliance, communication, etc.) which, though intertwined, have contributed separate elements to the final perception of the patient as a subjective body. The result is that the patient can no longer be encapsulated in a single gaze; the whole person is a multi-dimensional rather than unitary being.

The investing of the body and its relationship with a new mechanism of power has served to construct a novel range of medical problems and direct the medical gaze to new areas of concern; and, at these various points, new or revitalised medical specialties have been crystallised. In other words, it is neither the prior existence of a corpus of knowledge that allows 'professionalisation' in some areas, nor the imperialist construction of an ideology that serves professional ends, which explains the mutual interdependence of medical knowledge and the profession of medicine, but the subtle yet pervasive relationship of the body to a mechanism of power in the form of a system of surveillance.

The manifestations of the relationship between knowledge of the body and the power that invests it can also be seen in the emergence of many of the so-called paramedical occupations. The latter part of the twentieth century has witnessed an expansion in those health workers employed in community work or the promotion of positive health (rather than simply disease prevention). The history of health visitors or of health educators, for example, is another history of the extension of a disciplinary apparatus. Health educators who, two decades ago, wrote of the effects of telling people to stop smoking, are now engaged in writing up research which involves asking people for their individual reasons and rationale for smoking.

The new political anatomy of the body can be seen in the institutionalised mechanisms of surveillance which have emerged in the last few decades: the welfare state, the national health service, the current faith in 'community care'. It can also be seen in other non-medical areas such as educational theories, techniques and institutions; in parole, probation, open prisons, and community service; in the new techniques and surveillance possibilities of telecommunications which, as they inexorably extend themselves, evince an outcry against their threat to a privacy which, in a sense, they themselves have created.

Yet while the extended gaze of the Dispensary and survey have grown during the twentieth century, the Panopticon has not disappeared. Prisons, schools, workshops and hospitals are still built and used: indeed, with the growth in medical technology and super-specialties, the panoptic gaze has focused on an even more detailed analysis of the body. Thus, at the same time as the community gaze constructs identities and relationships, the Panopticon produces ever more discrete and individualised bodies. At times it is possible to detect areas of conflict or potential conflict between these two regimes, such as between hospital and community care, specialist versus generalist service, or the struggle for control of childbirth between hospital obstetrics and community childbirth alliances.[73]

But at another level it is important to see these various manifestations of conflict themselves as the product of a particular mechanism of power and its accompanying regime of truth. We must, as Foucault suggests, start the analysis where power is 'capillary ... in its more regional and local forms and institutions . . . at the more extreme point of its exercise'.[74] It is at these points that we can see power in immediate relationship with its field of application, and where it produces its real effects. It is in this context that the human body at the end of the eighteenth century enters 'a machinery of power that explores it, breaks it down and rearranges it. A "political anatomy", which was also a "mechanics of power", was being born.'[75] In the twentieth century the human body has been subjected to a more complex, yet perhaps more efficient, machinery of power which, from the moment of birth (or, more correctly, from the time of registration at an ante-natal clinic) to death, has constructed a web of investigation, observation and recording around individual bodies, their relationships and their subjectivity, in the name of health.

12

Postscript: the human sciences

The extension of a disciplinary apparatus throughout society at the end of the eighteenth century marked the emergence of a new power, a new knowledge and a new conception of the body. 'The moment that saw the transition from historico–ritual mechanisms for the formation of individuality to the scientifico–disciplinary mechanisms, when the normal took over from the ancestral, and measurement from status, thus substituting for the individuality of the memorable man that of the calculable man, that moment when the sciences of man became possible is the moment when a new technology of power and a new political anatomy of the body were implemented.'[1] The sciences of man – both biological and human – are therefore separate components of an overall apparatus of power which has as its object and its effect a particular political anatomy.

At the beginning of the twentieth century the Dispensary gaze transformed a physical space between individual bodies into a social one; at the same moment Emile Durkheim, the architect of the primacy of the social, was appointed to the first chair in the new discipline of sociology. These events are of course not mere coincidents but reflect the development and deployment in the human sciences of a pervasive gaze to the social, parallel to that of the medical sciences.

In the early decades of the century, for example, psychology played a major role in opening up the mind of everyone to surveillance, in promulgating regimes of mental hygiene, in refining theories of the neuroses and in creating techniques for explaining and measuring social relationships. There were undoubtedly many times during the inter-war years when it would have been possible to observe simultaneously a patient lying on the psychoanalyst's couch or sitting in the GP's surgery simply talking about themselves, while a sociologist of the 'Chicago school' was observing the everyday behaviour of people on the street or an anthropologist who supported the new techniques of field studies was silently noting the daily routines of some far-off tribe. Throughout society, social interaction and social space became an object of scrutiny and the confession, which had been the province of those who demanded secrets, truth and repentance, was deployed to gain access to the ordinary and the trivial.

The gaze commenced with the child. Psychologists played an important part in the discovery of the normal child, in revealing the detailed stages of child development, in classifying behaviour problems and in developing techniques of educational surveillance and child rearing. Sociologists, in their exploration of the social world of the child, discovered 'socialisation' and thereby transformed what had been seen exclusively as a biological trajectory into a social process.

Sociology made its principal contribution in the post-war world when its mastery of survey techniques made it of value to a medical gaze intent on exploring the surveillance possibilities of this newly discovered technology. Sociologists, in close alliance with medicine, opened up areas of the health experiences of 'ordinary' people through surveys of health attitudes, of illness behaviour, of drug taking and of symptom prevalence.

More recently, as the medical gaze has focused on individual idiosyncrasies, personal meanings and subjectivity, sociology too has turned its attention to fresh possibilities. On the one hand, various survey techniques have been made more sophisticated so that they might take into consideration, bring out or measure, individual meanings; on the other hand, some sociologists have explicitly rejected survey techniques on the grounds that they objectify respondents and have instead turned to methodologies which, they hold, more clearly respect or enhance patient subjectivity. Proponents of interaction analysis, participant observations, ethnomethodology, and other more naturalistic methods have, within the last decade, been critical of the dehumanising aspects of medicine and of sociology itself; and yet the effect of their stance is to have strengthened the power of gaze of the new medicine to the essentially subjective.

In psychiatry, sociology has provided a rich and diverse contribution to the extension of the medical gaze. Methodologically, it has offered psychiatry various techniques for the exploration of the mental functioning of individuals, ranging from the survey to participant observation; theoretically it, together with psychology, has helped to define basic concepts, such as stress and coping, which have enabled psychiatry to focus with ever-greater penetration on individual functioning. In short, sociology has reinforced the shift of the psychiatric gaze from arbitrary external referrents to internal subjective ones.

In general practice, behavioural scientists have helped in the discovery of 'minor morbidity' through survey techniques; they have promoted the visibility of the patient by investigating patient attitudes and behaviour; they have participated in the study of the organisation of care, of health centres and health care teams, so assisting the extension of the gaze. Sociologists have supported geriatricians in presenting the problem of chronic illness as a product of a recent change in the spectrum of morbidity in the community rather than as an invention of the gaze; and they have furthered the efficiency of this invention by promoting the study of the many social implications of chronic illness. In epidemiological studies of many different medical problems, sociologists have been brought in to help realise a wider multi-factorial aetiology in which social factors and environment play an important role. Many of the statistical and methodological techniques developed by sociologists have further been used in epidemiological investigations.

In a sense, these many examples are a somewhat arbitrary selection of points of contact between medicine and the human sciences; in reality, medicine and these sciences have been engaged in the same enterprise – the production of a discourse on the individual which corresponds to an extended disciplinary power. At the same moment as the patient entered medical discourse as a subject, he appeared in a parallel discourse in the human sciences; indeed, the changes in medical discourse often preceded those of the sociological discourse.

When Parsons wrote about the doctor–patient relationship in the context of the sick-role, in 1951, he was reflecting a contemporary medical concern with the respective roles of doctor and patient. He even specifically condoned, on theoretical grounds, a relatively passive role for the patient.[2] It is interesting to note that Brackenbury, sixteen years earlier, in his book of 1935 on the doctor–patient relationship, identified two of Parson's classic characteristics of the patient's role, obedience to the doctor and the will to get well.[3] Similarly when Freidson, in 1961, challenged this formulation and argued that there were objective differences in perspective between physician and patient and consequently conflicts of interest, he was merely expressing in sociological discourse what had already begun to be, and was continuing to be, debated in contemporary medical literature.[4] Again, Szasz & Hollender's 1956 formulation of the doctor–patient relationship, as ranging from activity–passivity to mutual cooperation,[5] appeared at the same time as Balint was writing of the same notions.[6] And Freidson's additions to the Szasz–Hollander typology, in 1970[7] (when he argued that the patient might be active and the doctor passive), came some four years after Browne & Freeling had pointed out how the patient could manipulate the doctor.[8]

Writing in 1975, Stimson & Webb[9] agreed with Rubington & Weinberg's claim, of 1968, that even medical sociology had tended to treat the patient as 'objectively given' rather than as 'subjectively problematic'.[10] 'We have', concluded Stimson & Webb, 'few accounts of the experience of the patient as a person.'[11] In effect, the elaboration of patient meanings in 'every-day medical settings'[12] had become the core of the medical sociological enterprise during the 1970s, at the same time as the various disciplines of the survey focused increasingly on the same object.

This is not to argue that the human sciences have simply been the handmaiden of medicine: their frequent alliances, points of contact and shared concerns do not reflect a relationship of domination but of a common object, namely, the body and its relationships, and a common effect, the subjectivity of that same body. The human sciences have thus produced an often independent but parallel gaze to the body and within this independence have forged a new 'regime of truth.' This knowledge has increasingly been concerned with the subjectivity of experience and has often sought to conceal its invention through the notion of alienation by presenting subjectivity as the immanent human condition which the human sciences have succeeded in 'liberating'.

In a paper published in 1976, Jewson argued that the 'sick-man' – that being predicated on the idiosyncratic personal experience of the patient – disappeared from 'medical cosmologies' between 1770 and 1870.[13] Specifically, he argued that the advent of pathological medicine at the end of the eighteenth century resulted in the prevailing 'person orientated cosmology' being usurped by an 'object' orientated one. Writing in 1977, Figlio also saw developments in this period as producing a form of 'medical alienation and reification: people losing a sense of wholeness, inviolability and ethical judgement'.[14] This suggests that the discovery of the patient in the medical and human sciences, during the last few decades, was in fact a rediscovery: that the sick-man had not so much appeared as reappeared. Yet these studies themselves belong to the human science discourse on the doctor–patient relationship of the 1970s. Perhaps Figlio's sub-title to his paper should be accepted for what it says: 'an invitation to the human sciences'.

The 'regime of truth' that the human sciences have produced involves an ethical polarisation of the subject–object relationship which privileges subjectivity as the form of moral autonomy.[15] It assumes that there already exists 'a human subject on the lines of the model provided by classical philosophy, endowed with a consciousness which power is then thought to seize on'.[16] Subjectivity might therefore be 'liberated' (by the humane social sciences) but it cannot be produced by domination; indeed, domination is held to falsify the very essence of human subjectivity. Hence, there has been an historical project in the human sciences which has concerned itself with the identification of a distant disappearance of 'a sense of wholeness, inviolability and ethical judgement' through forces of repression and domination which then enables claim to be made for the parallel *re*discovery and *re*appearance of the sick-man, by way of the human sciences. In effect, the recent social origins of the sick-man are blurred as a historical discourse on alienation provides him with a political credo, a universal status and a plausible history; an invention is translated into a language of liberation, a positive power which creates is concealed in the identification of a repressive power which is lifted. As Foucault points out, we continue to 'describe the effects of power in negative terms: it "excludes", it "represses", it "censors", it "abstracts", it "masks", it "conceals". In fact, power produces; it produces reality; it produces domains of objects and rituals of truth. The individual and the knowledge that may be gained of him belong to this production.'[17]

Political anatomy unifies those various sciences which have as their common object the human body and its surrounding space. In political anatomy those disparate knowledges, which have offered seemingly diverse or contradictory explanations of the body or its behaviour, can be seen as components of a single apparatus of power. The great debates of the twentieth century which oppose the individual and the social, the citizen and the State, the biological versus the environmental, are various manifestations of the same underlying dream, the same pervasive diagram of power. On the one hand, the social space around the body delimits and constrains it; on the other hand, it establishes, for the purposes of investigation, the reality of the individual as a social being who is able to manipulate that same social space. The techniques of surveillance are condemned as offending the individual freedoms that surveillance has fabricated; the right to private thoughts is celebrated, while, all around, those same thoughts are whispered in the great confession.

Power assumes knowledge and knowledge assumes power. It is only at the point where power plays on the body and its extended ontology that political anatomy is constructed. Perhaps, when Newton picked up a pebble from the beach and wondered about the great ocean of truth that lay all around him, his gaze did not veer from the pebble but fixed itself on the shadowy contours of a stone that had been fashioned by a multitude of elements.

Notes

Chapter 1

1 M. Foucault, *The birth of the clinic: an archeology of medical perception*, London, Tavistock, 1973.
2 *Ibid*, p. x.
3 M. Foucault, *Discipline and punish: the birth of the prison*, London, Allen Lane, 1977.
4 Unless otherwise referenced the other quotations in this chapter are from *ibid*, part III.
5 M. Foucault, *The history of sexuality*, vol. 1, London, Allen Lane, 1979, p. 94.

Chapter 2

1 H. Williams, *A century of public health in Britain*, London, Black, 1932, pp. 135–6.
2 S. Churchill, *Health services and the public*, London, Noel Douglas, 1928, p. 154.
3 H. Williams, *A century of public health*, p. 146.
4 M. Foucault, *The birth of the clinic: an archeology of medical perception*, London, Tavisock, 1973.
5 M. Foucault, *Discipline and punish: the birth of the prison*, London, Allen Lane, 1977, p. 198.
6 *Ibid*, p. 208.
7 See Donzelot for a parallel analysis of the invention of the social: J. Donzelot, *The policing of families*, London, Hutchison, 1979.
8 H. Williams, *Requiem for a great killer: the story of tuberculosis*, London, Health Horizon, 1973, p. 40.
9 E.W. Hope, *Textbook of public health*, Edinburgh, Livingstone, 1915.
10 H.W. Hill, *The new public health*, London, New York, Macmillan, 1916.
11 J.L. Burn, *Recent advances in public health*, London, Churchill, 1947.
12 H.W. Hill, *The new public health*, p. 17.
13 G. Newman, quoted in Editorial, *British Medical Journal*, vol. 2, 1920, p. 709.
14 R. Firth, reported in 'Report on Royal Sanitary Institute Congress', *British Medical Journal*, vol. 2, 1920, p. 212.
15 G. Newman, quoted in EDITORIAL, *British Medical Journal*, vol. 1, 1920, p. 646.
16 H. Williams, *Requiem for a great killer*, p. 39.
17 R.C. Wofinden, *Health services in England*, Bristol, John Wright, 1947, p. 71.
18 G. Bankoff, *The conquest of tuberculosis*, London, Macdonald, 1946, p. 162.

19 There had been a general interest in the venereal diseases, especially as they affected military efficiency and discipline, since the mid nineteenth century. By the twentieth century this interest had grown to be of more universal concern.

20 W.W. Jameson & F.T. Marchant, *A synopsis of hygiene*, London, Churchill, 1920, p. 187.

21 M. Morris, *The nation's health: the stamping out of venereal disease*, London, Cassel, 1917, p. 8.

22 B.A. Towers, 'Health education policy 1916–26: venereal disease and the prophylactic dilemma', *Medical History*, vol. 24, 1980, p. 70.

23 Reported in *British medical Journal*, vol. 2, 1930, p. 155.

24 Reported in *Lance*, vol. 1, 1926, p. 504.

25 Reported in *British Medical Journal*, vol. 2, 1930, p. 155.

26 *Ibid.*

27 Reported in *British Medical Journal*, vol.1, 1932, p. 536.

28 Reported in *British Medical Journal*, vol. 1, 1934, p. 958.

29 Reported in *British Medical Journal*, vol. 2, 1935, p. 343.

30 J.F. Goodhart, *The diseases of children*, London, 1885.

31 R. Hutchison *Lectures on diseases of children*, London, Arnold, 1904.

32 A. Garrod et al., *Diseases of children*, London, Arnold, 1913.

33 For history see A.W. Franklin, 'Paediatrics 1984', *Proceedings of the Royal Society of Medicine*, vol. 58, 1965, p. 392.

34 H. Cameron, *The nervous child*, London, Oxford University Press, 1919.

35 *Ibid*, p. v.

36 Board of Education, *Annual report for 1920 of the Chief Medical Officer*, London, HMSO, 1921, p. 109. Quoted in *The school health service: 1908–74*, London, HMSO, 1975.

37 The history of the early infant welfare movement is drawn from G.F. McCleary, *The maternity and child welfare movement*, London, King, 1935.

38 *Ibid.*

39 See, *The school health service: 1908–74.*

40 *Ibid*, p. 9.

41 *Ibid.*

42 Quoted in H. Williams, *Requiem for a great killer*, p. 33.

43 See, for example, E.W. Hope, *Textbook of public health* (9th edn), 1926.

44 *The school health service: 1908–74*, pp. 21–2.

45 Editorial, 'Hygiene in school', *Lancet*, vol. 2, 1926, p. 1173.

46 *The school health service: 1908–74*, p. 21.

47 See, for example, 'Joint meeting of Sections of Epidemiology and Medicine on air-conditioning', *Proceedings of the Royal Society of Medicine*, vol. 30, 1936–7, p. 1541.

48 J. Watt, 'Ventilation, heating and lighting of hospital wards', *Proceedings of the Royal Society of Medicine*, vol. 26, 1932–3, p. 1411.

49 *Ibid.*

50 W.A. Daley, 'Problems in hospital administration arising out of the Local Government Act, 1929', *Proceedings of the Royal Society of Medicine*, vol. 27, 1933–4, p. 1445.

51 J.A.H. Brinker, 'Convalescent homes of the future: their type, function and use', *Proceedings of the Royal Society of Medicine*, vol. 32, 1938–9, p. 369.
52 J.A.H. Brinker, 'Epidemiology applied to school life', *Lancet*, vol. 1, 1933, p. 569.
53 N. Jewson, 'Medical knowledge and the patronage system in 18th century England', *Sociology*, vol. 8, 1974, p. 369.
54 M. Foucault, *The Birth of the clinic.*
55 W. Hamer, 'The crux of epidemiology', *Proceedings of the Royal Society of Medicine*, vol. 24, 1930–1, p. 1425.

Chapter 3

1 L.C. Bruce, *Studies of clinical psychiatry*, London, Macmillan, 1906.
2 D.K. Henderson & R.D. Gillespie, *A textbook of psychiatry*, London, Oxford University Press, 1944 (6th edn).
3 M. Foucault, *Madness and civilization*, London, Tavistock, 1967.
4 *Ibid*, p. 246.
5 *Ibid*, p. 269.
6 M. Foucault, *Discipline and punish: the birth of the prison*, London, Allen Lane, 1977.
7 See, for example, K. Figlio, 'Chlorosis and chronic disease in 19th century Britain', *Social History*, vol. 3, 1978, p. 167.
8 The word neurosis was probably first used by Cullen in 1777 as a name for 'generalised affections of the nervous system': W. Cullen, *First lines of the practice of physic*, Edinburgh, 1777.
9 First diagnosed by Beard in 1880.
10 M. Craig, *Psychological medicine*, London, Churchill, 1905.
11 R.H. Cole, *Mental diseases*, London University Press, 1913.
12 M. Craig & T. Beaton, *Psychological medicine*, London, Churchill, 1926 (4th edn),
13 P. Stewart, *The diagnosis of nervous disease*, London, Edward Arnold, 1906.
14 H.C. Thompson, *Diseases of the nervous system*, London, Cassel, 1908.
15 P. Stewart, *The diagnosis of nervous disease*, p. 338.
16 W.H.B. Stoddart, *Mind and its disorders*, London, H.K. Lewis, 1908 (3rd edn: 1919).
17 *Ibid.*
18 R.H. Cole, *Mental diseases* (2nd edn: 1919), preface.
19 H.J. Norman, *Mental disorders for students and practitioners*, Edinburgh, Livingstone, 1928.
20 H. Devine, *Recent advances in psychiatry*, London, Churchill, 1929.
21 A. Cannon & E.D.T. Hayes, *The principles and practice of psychiatry*, London, Heinemann, 1932.
22 See, for example, Forsyth's (a general physician) paper on psychoanalysis, *Proceedings of the Royal Society of Medicine*, vol. 13, 1919–20.
23 P. Stewart, *The diagnosis of nervous disease* (6th edn: 1924), p. vii.
24 H.C. Thompson, *Diseases of the nervous system* (2nd edn: 1915; 3rd edn: 1921).
25 H. Rolleston, quoted in J.R. Lord, *The clinical study of mental disorders*, London, Adlard, 1926.
26 M.F. O'Hea, reported in *British Medical Journal*, vol. 1, 1928, p. 221.

27 E.F. Buzzard, 'The dumping ground of neurasthenia', *Lancet*, vol. 1, 1930, p. 1.
28 E.F. Buzzard, 'Medicine and the church', *Lancet*, vol. 2, 1927, p. 1007.
29 T.A. Ross, 'Morison Lectures', *Edinburgh Medical Journal*, vol. 42, 1935, p. 445.
30 Editorial, 'Psychotherapy by laymen', *Lancet*, vol. 1, 1939, p. 154.
31 'Annual report on medical education', *British Medical Journal*, vol. 2, 1920, p. 371.
32 'Annual report on medical education', *British Medical Journal*, vol. 2, 1921, p. 375.
33 'Annual report on medical education', *British Medical Journal*, vol. 2, 1922, p. 443.
34 D. Forsyth, 'The place of psychology in the medical curriculum', *Proceedings of the Royal Society of Medicine*, vol. 2, 1931–2, p. 1200.
35 'British Association annual meeting', *British Medical Journal*, vol. 2, 1928, p. 498.
36 Editorial, 'Psychology in the medical curriculum', *Lancet*, vol. 2, 1928, p. 559.
37 Editorial, 'Psychology in the medical curriculum', *British Medical Journal*, vol. 2, 1928, p. 539.
38 Editorial, 'Psychiatry for future doctors', *Lancet*, vol. 2, 1938, p. 1474.
39 This requirement was not, however, formalised in the GMC Recommendations until 1957.
40 *Royal Commission on Lunacy and Mental Disorder*, London, HMSO, 1926.
41 Editorial, 'The borderland of physiology and psychology', *Lancet*, vol. 1, 1928, p. 1023.
42 A. Meyer, 'The Maudsley Lecture', *Lancet*, vol. 1, 1933, p. 1129.
43 Editorial, 'Individual psychology', *British Medical Journal*, vol. 1, 1931, p. 148; and Editorial, 'Individual psychology', *Lancet*, vol. 1, 1931, p. 249.
44 W. Langdon-Brown, 'Applying knowledge to increase happiness', *Lancet*, vol. 1, 1933, p. 64.
45 W. Langdon-Brown, 'Individual psychology and the sympathetic mechanism', *British Medical Journal*, vol. 2, 1931, p. 753.
46 F.G. Crookshank, 'The psychological interest in general practice', *British Medical Journal*, vol. 1, 1932, *p*. 602.
47 H.V. Dicks, *Fifty years of the Tavistock Clinic*, London, Routledge and Kegan Paul, 1970.
48 H. Crichton-Miller, *Functional nerve disease*, London, Hodder and Stoughton, 1920, chapter 1; also H. Crichton-Miller, 'The physical basis of emotional disorder', *Proceedings of the Royal Society of Medicine*, vol. 17, 1923–4, p. 27.
49 H.V. Dicks, *Fifty years of the Tavistock Clinic.*
50 R.G. Gordon, N.G. Harris & J.R. Rees, *An introduction to psychological medicine*, London, Oxford University Press, 1936.
51 J.A. Ross, *The common neuroses*, London, Arnold, 1923.
52 H. Rolleston, quoted in *The clinical study of mental disorders.*
53 D. Forsyth, *Children in health and disease*, London, Murray, 1909.
54 J.C. McClure, 'Psychology and the practice of medicine', *British Medical Journal*, vol. 1, 1930, p. 610.
55 See next chapter for details of the Peckham experiment.
56 See, for example, Board of Education, *Report of the consultative committee on psychological tests of educable capacity and their possible use in the public system of education*, London, HMSO, 1924.

57 D. Armstrong, 'Child development and medical ontology', *Social Science and Medicine*, vol. 13, 1979, p. 9.
58 Editorial, 'National Institute of Child Psychology', *British Medical Journal*, vol. 2, 1931, p. 663.
59 D.R. MacCalman, 'The present status and functions of the child guidance movement in Great Britain and its possible future developments', *Journal of Mental Science*, vol. 85, 1939, p. 505.
60 H. Cameron, *The nervous child*, London, Oxford University Press, 1919.
61 Joint meeting of Section of Psychiatry and for Study of Disease in Children, 'The difficult child', *Proceedings of the Royal Society of Medicine*, vol. 23, 1929–30, p. 573.
62 Joint meeting, 'On eneuresis', *Proceedings of the Royal ociety of Medicine*, vol. 28, 1934–5.
63 A. Garrod et al. (eds.), *Diseases of children*, London, Arnold, 1913.
64 *The school health service 1908–74*, London, HMSO, 1975, p. 24.
65 *Ibid*, pp. 22, 24.
66 R. Hutchison, *Lectures on diseases of children*, London, Arnold, 1925 (5th edn).
67 *Ibid.*
68 H.V. Dicks, 'Principles of mental hygiene', in N.G. Harris (ed.), *Modern trends in psychological medicine: 1948*, London, Butterworth, 1948.
69 E.F. Buzzard, 'Some aspects of mental hygiene', *Proceedings of the Royal Society of Medicine*, vol. 14, 1920–1.
70 D.K. Henderson, quoted in Editorial, 'Social psychiatry', *Lancet*, vol. 2, 1931, p. 81.
71 H.V. Dicks, 'Principles of mental hygiene'.
72 M. Culpin, 'A Study of the incidence of the minor psychoses', *Proceedings of the Royal Society of Medicine*, vol. 21, 1927–8, p. 419.
73 M. Culpin, 'Occupational neuroses (including miners' nystagmus)', *Proceedings of the Royal Society of Medicine*, vol. 26, 1932–3, p. 655.
74 Editorial, 'Industrial hygiene', *British Medical Journal*, vol. 2, 1935, p. 1678.
75 R.F. Tredgold, 'Mental hygiene in industry', in *Modern trends in psychological medicine.*
76 D.K. Henderson, quoted in *Lancet* Editorials, 1931.
77 F.G. Crookshank, 'The psychological interest in general practice', *British Medical Journal*, vol. 1, 1932, p. 599.
78 J.C. McClure, 'Psychology and the practice of medicine', p. 610.
79 T.F. Rodger, 'Personnel selection', in *Modern trends in psychological medicine.*
80 Editorial, 'Psychiatry and the services', *Lancet*, vol. 1, 1940, p. 839.
81 *The works of psychologists and psychiatrists in the services*, London, HMSO, 1947.
82 J.C. McClure, 'Psychology and the practice of medicine'. p. 610.
83 'Annual medical education review', *British Medical Journal*, vol. 2, 1932, p. 479.
84 E. Glover, 'The birth of social psychiatry', *Lancet*, vol. 2, 1940, p. 239.
85 A.A.W. Petrie, 'History of psychiatric developments', *Journal of Mental Science*, vol. 91, 1945, p. 267.
86 Editorial, 'Intolerance in psychiatry', *Lancet*, vol. 2, 1931, p. 1089.
87 J.C. McClure, 'Psychology and the practice of medicine', p. 611.
88 Editorial, 'Expanding psychotherapy', *Lancet*, vol. 1, 1936, p. 1078.

89 M. Culpin, 'Psychology in medicine', *Lancet*, vol. 2, 1945, p. 519.
90 J.R. Lord, *The clinical study of mental disorders.*
91 M. Craig & T. Beaton, *Psychological medicine.*
92 R. Worth, 'Four decades of psychiatry', *Journal of Mental Science*, vol. 81, 1935, p. 755.
93 R.A. Noble, 'The place of psychology in medical education', *Journal of Mental Science*, vol. 78, 1932, p. 793.
94 H.V. Dicks, *Fifty years of the Tavistock Clinic.*
95 Editorial, 'Royal Medico-Psychological Association at Oxford', *British Medical Journal*, vol. 2, 1930, p. 69.
96 Editorial, 'Psychiatric clinic at Guy's', *Lancet*, vol. 1, 1939, p. 996.
97 Editorial, 'Psychiatry and general medicine', *Lancet*, vol. 2, 1942, p. 128.
98 Editorial, 'Psychiatric training', *Lancet*, vol. 2, 1943, p. 294.
99 R.H. Cole, *Mental diseases.*
100 D.K. Henderson & R.D. Gillespie, *A textbook of psychiatry.*
101 D.K. Henderson, reported in Editorial, 'Controversial ground in psychiatry', *Lancet*, vol. 1, 1939, p. 654.
102 Editorial, 'Research in psychiatry', *Lancet*, vol. 1, 1935, p. 1223.
103 D.K. Henderson, quoted in *Lancet* Editorial, 1939.

Chapter 4

1 Consultative Council on Medical and Allied Services, *Interim report on the future provision of medical and allied services* (Dawson Report), London, HMSO, 1920.
2 *Ibid*, para. 51.
3 *Ibid*, para. 90.
4 *Interdepartmental Committee on Insurance Medical Records* (Rolleston Report), London, HMSO, 1920. These issues are discussed by F. Honigsbaum, *The division in British medicine*, London, Kogan Page, 1979, p. 94.
5 Dawson report, para. 136.
6 *Ibid*, para. 137.
7 J.B. Atkins, *National physical training*, London, Isbister, 1904.
8 *Syllabus of physical training for schools*, London, Board of Education, 1909 and 1919.
9 *Ibid*, p. 4.
10 *Ibid*, pp. 8–10.
11 Dawson Report, para. 141.
12 Quoted in Editorial, 'Newman lecture on public health', *British Medical Journal*, vol. 1, 1920, p. 646.
13 Quoted in Editorial, 'Health through ministry', *British Medical Journal*, vol. 2, 1920, p. 709.
14 F. Honigsbaum, *The division in British medicine*, p. 147.
15 The 'Peckham experiment' led to a stream of publications. Two important books to emerge were: *Biologists in search of material: an interim report on the work of the Pioneer health centre, Peckham.* London, Faber and Faber, 1938; I.H. Pearse & L.H. Crocker, *The Peckham experiment: a study in the living structure of society*, London, George Allen and Unwin, 1943.

16 I.H. Pearse & L.H. Crocker, *The Peckham experiment*, p. 12.
17 *Ibid*, p. 13.
18 Annual report, *Pioneer health centre*, 1935–6, p. 9.
19 *Biologists in search of material*, p. 48.
20 Annual report, *Pioneer health centre*, 1935–6, p. 8.
21 I.H. Pearse & L.H. Crocker, *The Peckham experiment*, pp. 79–92.
22 *Biologists in search of material*, pp. 43–4.
23 I.H. Pearse & L.H. Crocker, *The Peckham experiment.*
24 J.M. Last, 'The iceberg: completing the clinical picture in general practice', *Lancet*, vol. 2, 1963, p. 28.
25 See, for example, D. Mechanic, 'The concept of illness behaviour', *Journal of Chronic Diseases*, vol. 15, 1962, p. 189.
26 Annual report, *Pioneer health centre*, 1935–6, p. 11.
27 I.H. Pearse & L.H. Crocker, *The Peckham experiment*, pp. 76–7.
28 *Ibid*, p. 68.
29 *Ibid*, p. 83.
30 J.A. Ryle, *Changing disciplines: lectures on the history, methods and motives of social pathology*, London, Oxford University Press, 1948, p. 1.
31 *Ibid*, p. 2.
32 *Ibid*, p. 4.
33 *Ibid*, p. 24.
34 Social and Preventive Medicine Committee of the Royal College of Physicians, *Interim report on the teaching of social and preventive medicine*, London, Royal College of Physicians, 1943.
35 *Ibid*, p. 3.
36 *Ibid*, pp. 13–15.
37 N.M. Goodman & C. Morris, 'The clinical teaching of social medicine', *Proceedings of the Royal Society of Medicine*, vol. 33, 1939–40, p. 751; also the discussion in *Proceedings of the Royal Society of Medicine*, vol. 37, 1943–4, p. 194.
38 *Report of the Inter-Departmental Committee on Medical Schools* (Goodenough Report), London, HMSO, 1944.
39 *Ibid*, p. 167.
40 *Ibid*, pp. 169–70.
41 M. Foucault, *Discipline and punish: the birth of the prison*, London, Allen Lane, 1977, p. 209.
42 F.A.E Crewe, 'Social medicine: an academic discipline and an instrument of social policy', *Lancet*, vol. 2, 1944, p. 618.
43 *Ibid.*
44 W. Jameson, 'War and the advancement of social medicine', *Lancet*, vol. 2, 1942, p. 479.
45 *Ibid.*

Chapter 5

1 W.P.D. Logan & E.M. Brooke, *Survey of Sickness, 1943–52*, London, HMSO, 1957, pp. 1–4. (These milestones of survey research were selected by Logan &

Brooke for their preliminary 'history' of survey techniques. Such histories, in tending to suggest the wisdom that follows, inevitably document progressive enlightenment.)

2 M. Foucault, *Discipline and punish: the birth of the prison*, London, Allen Lane, 1977.

3 *Ibid.*

4 T. Lewis, 'Research in medicine: its position and its needs', *British Medical Journal*, vol. 1, 1930, p. 479.

5 *Ibid*, p. 481.

6 *Ibid*, p. 480.

7 T. Lewis, 'Harveian oration on clinical science', *British Medical Journal*, vol. 2, 1933, p. 720.

8 *Ibid.*

9 T.I. Bennett & J.A. Ryle, 'Normal gastric function', *Guy's Hospital Reports*, vol. 71, 1921, p. 286.

10 J.A. Ryle, *Changing disciplines*, London, Oxford University Press, 1948, p. 70.

11 A.K. Shapiro, 'A contribution to a history of the placebo effect', *Behavioural Science*, vol. 5, 1960, p. 109.

12 *Ibid.*

13 Editorial, 'Amateur medical statisticians', *Lancet*, vol. 1, 1943, p. 19.

14 Editorial, 'Patulin disappoints', *Lancet*, vol. 2, 1944, p. 380.

15 As judged by A. Cochrane, 'The random controlled trial', *Lancet*, vol. 1, 1972, p. 985.

16 Medical Research Council, 'Streptomycin treatment of tuberculous meningitis', *Lancet*, vol. 1, 1948, p. 582.

17 Medical Research Council, 'Streptomycin treatment of pulmonary tuberculosis', *British Medical Journal*, vol. 2, 1948, p. 769.

18 Editorial, 'The controlled therapeutic trial', *British Medical Journal*, vol. 2, 1948, p. 796.

19 Editorial, 'Streptomycin in pulmonary tuberculosis', *Lancet*, vol. 2, 1948, p. 733.

20 This section draws on a previous paper: D. Armstrong, 'Clinical sense and clinical science', *Social Science and Medicine*, vol. 11, 1977, p. 599.

21 Editorial, 'Mathematics and medicine', *Lancet*, vol. 1, 1937, p. 31.

22 A.B. Hill, *Principles of medical statistics*, London, *The Lancet*, 1937.

23 M. Greenwood & W.W.C. Topley, 'Experimental epidemiology: some general considerations', *Proceedings of the Royal Society of Medicine*, vol. 19, 1925–6, p. 31.

24 *Ibid.*

25 See, for example, W. Hamer, 'The crux of epidemiology', *Proceedings of the Royal Society of Medicine*, vol. 24, 1930–1, p. 1425.

26 J.E. Lane-Clayton, *A further report on cancer of the breast with special reference to its associated antecedent conditions*, London, HMSO, 1926.

27 R. Doll & A.N. Hill, 'Smoking and cancer of the lung', *British Medical Journal*, vol. 2, 1950, p. 739.

28 W. Pickles, 'Epidemiology in country practice', *Proceedings of the Royal Society of Medicine*, vol. 28, 1934–5, p. 1337.

29 B.E. Spear & C.A. Gould 'Mechanical tabulation of hospital records', *Proceedings of the Royal Society of Medicine*', vol. 30, 1936–7, p. 633.
30 J.A. Ryle, *Changing disciplines.*
31 P. Stocks, 'The measurement of morbidity', *Proceedings of the Royal Society of Medicine*, vol. 37, 1943–4, p. 59.
32 J.A. Ryle, *Changing disciplines.*
33 *Ibid.*
34 W.P.D. Logan & E.M. Brooke, *Survey of Sickness.*
35 Annual report of the Chief Medical Officer, *On the state of the public health*, London, Ministry of Health, 1920, p. 137.
36 *Ibid* (1924).
37 *Ibid* (1931).
38 *Ibid* (1935).
39 *Ibid.*
40 See chapter 4 of this book.
41 T. Jeffery, 'Mass Observation', paper presented to Annual Conference of the Society for the Social History of Medicine, 1980.
42 W. Langdon-Brown, quoted at conference on 'The social environment and the war', *Lancet*, vol. 1, 1940, p. 285.
43 K. Box & G. Thomas, 'The War-time Social Survey', *Journal of the Royal Statistical Society*, vol. 107, 1944, p. 151.
44 Details reported in *Lancet*, vol. 2, 1940, p. 144.
45 *Ibid.*
46 K. Box & G. Thomas, 'War-time Social Survey', p. 151.
47 Editorial, 'Results of the War-time Social Survey', *Lancet*, vol. 2, 1940, p. 305.
48 Report of the Chief Medical OffiCER, *On the state of the public health during six years of war*, London, HMSO, 1946, p. 118.
49 *Ibid.*
50 K. Box & G. Thomas, 'War-time Social Survey', p. 177.
51 D. MacKay, *Hospital morbidity statistics.* Studies on Medical and Population Subjects, no. 4, London, HMSO, 1951.
52 Reported in W.P.D. Logan & E.M. Brooke, *Survey of Sickness*, p. 12.
53 Editorial, 'A health survey', *Lancet*, vol. 1, 1944, p. 829.
54 P. Stocks, The measurement of morbidity.
55 J.A. Ryle, *Changing disciplines*, pp. 79–81.
56 J.A. Ryle, *Changing disciplines*, p. 82.
57 K. Box & G. Thomas, 'War-time Social Survey', p. 177.
58 J.A. Ryle, *Changing disciplines.*
59 K. Box & G. Thomas, 'War-time Social Survey', pp. 55–64.
60 J.A. Ryle, *Changing disciplines*, pp. 55–64.
61 C. Gordon (ed.), *Michel Foucault: power/knowledge*, Brighton, Harvester, 1980.
62 K. Box & G. Thomas, 'War-time Social Survey', p. 153.
63 Editorial, 'Sample surveys', *Lancet*, vol. 2, 1950, p. 22.
64 M. Foucault, *Discipline and punish: the birth of the prison*, London, Allen Lane, 1977.
65 J.A. Ryle, *Changing disciplines*, p. 64.

Chapter 6

1 The various sociological analyses of the medical profession, which have emerged in the post-war years, from functionalist to Marxist, can all be seen to have struggled with the relationship between the profession and power though even at its most explicit the role of power has been subsidiary. See, for example, T.J. Johnson, *Professions and power*, London, Macmillan, 1972.

2 R. Stevens, *Medical practice in modern England: the impact of specialisation and state medicine*, New Haven, Yale, 1966; R. Bucher & A. Strauss, 'Professions in process', *American Journal of Sociology*, vol. 66, 1961, p. 325.

3 Cohen, for example, suggested that during the last few decades 'speialities have arisen which are based on vastly diverse criteria': H. Cohen, 'Reflections on specialisation in medicine', *Annals of the Royal College of Surgeons*, vol. 27, 1960 p. 1.

4 See chapter 2 of this book.

5 This chapter is partly based on D. Armstrong, 'Child development and medical ontology', *Social Science and Medicine*, vol. 13, 1979, p. 9.

6 Various textbooks on diseases of children had been published; at Great Ormond Street a Hospital for Sick Children had been opened. See chapter 2 of this book.

7 D. Forsyth, *Children in health and disease*, London, John Murray, 1909, p. 271.

8 R. Hutchison, 'Paediatrics, present and prospective', *Lancet*, vol. 2, 1940, p. 799.

9 See chapter 3 of this book.

10 *Archives of Disease in Childhood*, founded in 1924, was the journal of the British Paediatric Association.

11 D. Jameson, 'Effects of war-time rationing on child health', *Proceedings of the Royal Society of Medicine*, vol. 35, 1941–2, p. 273.

12 Quoted at meeting of Section for Study of Disease in Childhood on 'School medical services – present and future', *Proceedings of the Royal Society of Medicine*, vol. 38, 1944–5, p. 373.

13 Discussions published in *Proceedings of the Royal Society of Medicine*, 1939–45.

14 Discussion on 'Effects of war-time rationing on child health', *Proceedings of the Royal Society of Medicine*, vol. 35, 1941–2, p. 273.

15 Discussion on 'Nutritional anaemia in children and women: a war-time problem', *Proceedings of the Royal Society of Medicine*, vol. 36, 1942–3, p. 69.

16 *Ibid.*

17 Reported in discussion on 'Decline in breast feeding', *Proceedings of the Royal Society of Medicine*, vol. 36, 1942–3, p. 382.

18 'Nutritional survey of school children in Oxfordshire, London and Birmingham', *Proceedings of the Royal Society of Medicine*, vol. 37, 1943–4, p. 313.

19 Reported at British Paediatric Association AGM, *Archives of Disease in Childhood*, vol. 24, 1949. See note 25.

20 G.M. Allen-Williams, 'Some observations on the growth of children', *Archives of Disease in Childhood*, vol. 21, 1946, p. 190.

21 R.W.P. Ellis, 'Height and weight in relation to onset of puberty in boys', *Archives of Disease in Childhood*, vol. 21, 1946, p. 181.

22 C. Asher, 'The relationship of birth weight to mental development', *Archives of Disease in Childhood*, vol. 23, 1948, p. 142.
23 F. Faulkner, 'Measurement in growth and development studies', *Archives of Disease in Childhood*, vol. 27, 1952, p. 303.
24 R.C. MacKeith, 'Measurement and the paediatrician', *Developmental Medicine and Child Neurology*, vol. 6, 1964, p. 453.
25 The MRC Survey under Douglas took its cohort from 1948. Early results were published in the 1950s, the results of the Ministry of Health Survey in 1959: *Standards of Normal Weight in Infancy.* Reports on Public Health and Medical Subjects, no. 99, London, HMSO, 1959.
26 E.R. Bransby, quoted in the 'Report of the Height and Weight Survey Sub-Committee of the British Paediatric Association', *Archives of Disease in Childhood*, vol. 19, 1944, p. 37.
27 E.R. Brandsby & W.H. Hammon, 'Growth and development standards and their clinical application', *Proceedings of the Royal Society of Medicine*, vol. 43, 1950, p. 825.
28 J.M. Tanner, *ibid*, p. 824.
29 J.W.B. Douglas, *ibid*, p. 828.
30 R.S. Illingworth, *The normal child*, London, Churchill, 1953.
31 *Ibid* (2nd edn: 1957), p. v.
32 *Ibid.* (3rd edn: 1964), p. 196.
33 J. Apley, 'Paediatrics and the undergraduate curriculum', *Lancet*, vol. 2, 1965, p. 633.
34 Editorial, 'Growth in childhood', *British Medical Journal*, vol. 1, 1957, p. 1232.
35 Editorial, 'Environment and heredity', *British Medical Journal*, vol. 1, 1950, p. 887.
36 Editorial, 'The growth and development of children', *British Medical Journal*, vol. 1, 1952, p. 963.
37 Reported at the British Paediatric Association AGM, *Archives of Disease in Childhood*, vol. 18, 1943, p. 54.
38 'Report of Child Psychology Sub-Committee of the British Paediatric Association', *Archives of Disease in Childhood*, vol. 22, 1946, p. 57.
39 Reported in *Archives of Disease in Childhood*, vol. 23, 1948, p. 141.
40 Particularly, A. Gesell et al., *Biographies of child development: the mental growth and careers of 84 infants and children*, London, Hamish Hamilton, 1939.
41 For history see A. Gesell, *Infant behaviour: its genesis and growth*, New York, McGraw-Hill, 1934.
42 A. Gesell et al., *Biographies of child development.*
43 For details see A. Gesell, *Infant and child in the culture of today: the guidance of development in home and nursery school*, London, Hamish Hamilton, 1943.
44 A. Gesell, *The pre-school child from the standpoint of public hygiene and education*, Cambridge, Mass., 1923.
45 A. Gesell et al., *Biographies of child development.* p. 309.
46 A.W. Franklin, 'Paediatrics 1984', *Lancet*, vol. 1, 1965, p. 117.
47 *Ibid.*
48 B. Corner, 'Progress in perinatal paediatrics', *Proceedings of the Royal Society of Medicine*, vol. 57, 1964, p. 231.

49 N.B. Capon, 'The training of clinical teachers', *Proceedings of the Royal Society of Medicine*, vol. 39, 1945–6, p. 65.
50 Editorial, 'More paediatric planning', *Lancet*, vol. 2, 1942, p. 370.
51 G.B. Fleming, 'Why not an adolescents' hospital?', *Lancet*, vol. 1, 1942, p. 631.
52 P. Catzel, 'Paediatrics', *British Medical Journal*, vol. 2, 1955, p. 1028.
53 J. Apley, 'Paediatrics and the undergraduate curriculum'.
54 R.G. Mitchell, 'The community paediatrician', *British Medical Journal*, vol. 2, 1971, p. 95.
55 R.G. Mitchell, 'The child, science and society', *Lancet*, vol. 1, 1964, p. 181.
56 'Report of the Executive Committee of the British Paediatric Association', *Archives of Disease in Childhood*, vol. 35, 1960, p. 412.
57 'Report of the Nursing Committee of the British Paediatric Association', *Archives of Disease in Childhood*, vol. 40, 1965, p. 448.
58 R.G. Mitchell, 'The child, science and society'.
59 Report of the Committee on Child Health Services, *Fit for the future*, London, HMSO, 1976.
60 S.D.M. Court & A. Jackson, *Paediatrics in the seventies*, London, Nuffield Provincial Hospitals Trust, 1972.
61 Report of the Committee on Child Health Services.
62 A.W. Franklin, 'Paediatrics 1984'.
63 J. Apley, 'Paediatrics and the undergraduate curriculum'.
64 S.D.M. Court, 'Child health in a changing community', *British Medical Journal*, vol. 1, 1971, p. 125.
65 M.A. Salmon, 'Developmental paediatrics', *Lancet*, vol. 1, 1972, p. 379.
66 N.B. Capon, 'Development and behaviour of children', *British Medical Journal*, vol. 1, 1950, p. 859.
67 R.S. Illingworth, *The normal child*, preface.
68 *Ibid*, p. 89.
69 *Ibid*, p. 216.

Chapter 7

1 *Report of the Mental Deficiency Committee*, London, HMSO, 1929; see p. 2 for a description of the history of the report.
2 *Ibid*, p. 1.
3 *Ibid*, p. 3.
4 *Ibid*, p. 3.
5 E.O. Lewis, *Report on an investigation into the incidence of mental deficiency in six areas, 1925–1927*, London, HMSO, 1929.
6 The Mental Deficiency Act of 1913 required all mentally defective children to be known; the Elementary Education (Defective and Epileptic Children) Act of 1914 further required that they should receive appropriate education.
7 E.O. Lewis, *Mental deficiency*, p. 22.
8 P. Lemkau et al., 'A survey of statistical studies on the prevalence and incidence of mental disorder in sample populations', *Public Health Reports*, vol. 58, 1943, p. 1909.

9 E. Slater, 'The incidence of mental disorder', *Annals of Eugenics, vol.* 6, 1934–5, p. 172.
10 E. Slater, 'A demographic study of a psychopathic population', *Annals of Eugenics,* vol. 12, 1943–5, p. 121.
11 W. Mayer-Gross, 'Mental health survey in a rural area: a preliminary report', *Eugenics Review,* vol. 40, 1948–9, p. 141.
12 *Ibid,* p. 140.
13 *Ibid.*
14 E. Glover, 'The birth of social psychiatry', *Lancet,* vol. 2, 1940, p. 239.
15 *Ibid.*
16 H. Devine, *Recent advances in psychiatry,* London, Churchill, 1929.
17 Editorial, 'The prognosis of schizophrenia', *Lancet,* vol. 1, 1938, p. 384.
18 Editorial, 'Insulin in schizophrenia', *Lancet,* vol. 1, 1936, p. 1418.
19 A.T. Scull, *Decarceration: community treatment and the deviant,* Englewood Cliffs, Prentice-Hall, 1977.
20 See, for example, K. Jones, *A history of the mental health services,* London, Routledge and Kegan Paul, 1972.
21 Editorial, 'The psychiatric day hospital', *Lancet,* vol. 1, 1955, p. 442.
22 Editorial, 'Visiting in mental hospitals', *Lancet,* vol. 1, 1956, p. 334.
23 Editorial, 'Walls of Jericho', *Lancet,* vol. 1, 1957. p. 1177.
24 M. Culpin, 'Psychology in medicine', *Lancet,* vol. 2, 1945, p. 519.
25 F.M.R. Walshe, *Diseases of the nervous system,* London, Edinburgh, Livingstone, 1908.
26 Editorial, 'Brain and mind', *Lancet,* vol. 2, 1947. p. 357.
27 W.R. Brain, *Diseases of the nervous system,* London, Oxford University Press, 1933.
28 Editorial, 'The biological approach to mental disorder', *Lancet,* vol. 1, 1941, p. 544.
29 H.M. Flanagan, 'In the mental hospital', *Lancet,* vol. 2, 1955, p. 1295.
30 H. Merskey & W.L. Tonge, *Psychiatric illness,* London, Bailliere Tindall, 1965, p. 15.
31 J.G. Howells, *Nosology of psychiatry,* London, Society of Clinical Psychiatrists, 1970.
32 S. Crown, *Essential principles of psychiatry,* London, Pitman, 1970.
33 M. Hamilton (ed.), *Fish's clinical psychopathology,* Bristol, John Wright, 1974.
34 W.H. Trethowen, *Psychiatry,* London, Bailliere Tindall, 1979, p. 97.
35 *Memorandum on the Future Organisation of Psychiatric Services,* Jointly produced by the Royal College of Physicians, the BMA group of practitioners of psychological medicine and the Royal Medico–Psychological Association, 1945.
36 F. Fish, 'Psychiatry as a medical specialty', *Lancet,* vol. 1, 1965, p. 565.
37 See, for example, L. Srole et al., *Mental health in the metropolis: the midtown study,* New York, McGraw-Hill, 1962; and D.C. Leighton et al., *The character of danger,* New York, Free Press, 1963.
38 E.J.R. Primrose, *Psychological illness: a community study,* London, Tavistock, 1962; G.W. Brown & T. Harris, *Social origins of depression,* London, Tavistock, 1979.

39 See chapter 8 of this book.
40 See, for example, M. Balint, *The doctor, his patient and the illness*, London, Pitman, 1957.
41 R.F. Tredgold, 'The integration of psychiatric teaching in the curriculum', *Lancet*, vol. 1, 1962, p. 1345.
42 F. Fish, 'Psychiatry as a medical specialty', p. 567.
43 R.F. Tredgold, 'The integration of psychiatric teaching'.
44 Editorial, 'Teaching psychiatry', *Lancet*, vol. 1, 1961, p. 814.
45 *Royal Commission on Medical Education*, London, HMSO, 1968.
46 D.K. Henderson & R.D. Gillespie, *A textbook of psychiatry*, London, Oxford University Press, 1944 (6th edn).
47 T.S. Clouston, *Unsoundness of mind*, London, Methuen, 1911, p. 322.
48 J.A. Ross, *The common neuroses*, London, Edward Arnold, 1923.
49 I. Skottowe, 'Psychological medicine: current methods of treatment', *Lancet*, vol. 1, 1944, p. 329.
50 M. Jones & R.N. Rapoport, 'Administrative and social psychiatry', *Lancet*, vol. 2, 1955, p. 386.
51 D.H. Clark, 'Administrative therapy', *Lancet*, vol. 1, 1958, p. 805.
52 J.A.R. Bickford, 'The forgotten patient', *Lancet*, vol. 2, 1955, p. 969.
53 D.V. Martin, 'Institutionalisation', *Lancet*, vol. 2, 1955, p. 1188. There is also the large sociological literature. See especially E. Goffman, *Asylums: essays on the social situation of mental patients and other in-mates*, London, Penguin, 1961.
54 A. Lewis, 'Between guesswork and certainty in psychiatry', *Lancet*, vol. 1, 1958, p. 173.
55 D.R. MacCalman, 'The development of psychiatry within the NHS', *Proceedings of the Royal Society of Medicine*, vol. 42, 1949, p. 365.
56 D. Curran, 'Psychiatry united', *Proceedings of the Royal Society of Medicine*, vol. 45, 1951–2, p. 105.
57 See, for example, T. Szasz, *The myth of mental illness*, London, Paladin, 1961; R. Boyers & R. Orrill, *Laing and anti-psychiatry*, London, Penguin, 1972.
58 S. Crown, 'Essential principles of psychiatry', p. 19.
59 R.F. Tredgold, 'The integration of psychiatric teaching'.
60 W.H. Trethowen, *Psychiatry*, p. 54.
61 Ibid, p. 52.
62 D. Curran, M. Partridge & P. Storey, *Psychological medicine*, London, Churchill Livingstone, 1972, p. 68 also R.E. Kendell, *The role of diagnosis in psychiatry*, Oxford, Blackwell, 1975.
63 M. Bleuler, quoted in D. Hill, 'The bridge between neurology and psychiatry', *Lancet*, vol. 1, 1964, p. 513.
64 Jasper's *General psychopathology* was translated by Hamilton, published in 1963, and proved influential. See, for example, F.K. Taylor, *Psychopathology: its causes and symptoms*, London, 1966; or D. Bannister, 'Repertory grid technique', *British Journal of Psychiatry*, vol. 3, 1965, p. 977.
65 D. Curran et al. *Psychological medicine* (5th edn onwards).
66 H. Merskey & W.L. Tonge, *Psychiatric illness*, p. 21.
67 *Ibid*, p. 6.

Chapter 8

1 M. Foucault, *Discipline and punish: the birth of the prison*, London, Allen Lane, 1977, see part III; also chapter 1 of this book.
2 R. Pinker, *English hospital statistics: 1861–1938*, London, Heinemann, 1966.
3 Editorial, 'The renaissance of general practice', *Lancet*, vol. 2, 1929, p. 933.
4 A.G. Signy, 'Trends in clinical pathologists', *Journal of Clinical Pathology*, vol. 23, 1970, p. 744.
5 Editorial, 'Clinical specialism', *Lancet*, vol. 2, 1945, p. 209.
6 B. Moynihan, reported under 'Medical news', *Lancet*, vol. 2, 1929, p. 957.
7 Editorial, 'General practitioners and hospitals', *British Medical Journal*, vol. 2, 1949, p. 1031.
8 O.R. Tisdall, 'The general practitioner and scientific thought', *British Medical Journal*, vol. 1, 1941, p. 722.
9 H. Crichton-Miller, 'Training of the general practitioner', *Lancet*, vol. 2, 1945, p. 231.
10 Editorial 'Research in general practice', *Lancet*, vol. 2, 1926, p. 863.
11 *Ibid.*
12 C. Lindsay, 'The profession and the public', *British Medical Journal*, vol. 2, 1938, p. 163.
13 H.H. Sanguinetti, 'A general practitioner service', *British Medical Journal*, vol. 1, 1942, p. 25.
14 *Lancet*, Editorial, 'Research in general practice'.
15 See, for an overview, R.J.F.H. Pinsent, 'James MacKenzie and research tomorrow', *Journal of the College of General Practitioners*, vol. 190, 1963, p. 114.
16 W. Pickles, *Epidemiology in a country practice*, Bristol, Wright, 1939.
17 W. Pickles, 'Epidemiology in the Yorkshire Dales', *Practitioner*, vol. 74, 1955, p. 76.
18 Pointed out by F. Honigsbaum, *The division in British medicine*, London, Frank Page, 1979.
19 Editorial, 'Psychotherapy in general practice', *Lancet*, vol. 1, 1939, p. 707.
20 C. Lindsay, 'The profession and the public', p. 164.
21 Editorial, 'The Presidential address', *British Medical Journal*, vol. 2, 1938, p. 183.
22 P. Stocks, *Sickness in the population of England and Wales: 1844–47*, London, HMSO, 1949.
23 J. Pemberton, 'Illness in general practice', *British Medical Journal*, vol. 1, 1949, p. 306.
24 R.M. McGregor, 'The work of a family doctor', *Edinburgh Medical Journal*, vol. 57, 1950, p. 433.
25 J. Fry, 'A year of general practice: a study in morbidity', *British Medical Journal*, vol. 2, 1952, p. 429.
26 T.S. Kuhn, *The structure of scientific revolutions*, Chicago University Press, 1962.
27 J. Fry, 'A year of general practice'.
28 Logan, W.P.D. *General practitioner's records: an analysis of the clinical records of 8 practices during the period April 1951–March 1952*, London, HMSO, 1953.

29 *Measurement of morbidity*, London, HMSO, 1954.
30 W.P.D. Logan & E.M. Brooke, *The survey of Sickness, 1943–52*, London, HMSO, 1957.
31 W.P.D. Logan & A.A. Cushion, *Morbidity statistics from general practice*, vol. 1, London, HMSO, 1958.
32 Editorial, 'The Morbidity Survey – and after', *Journal of the College of General Practitioners*, vol. 2, 1959, p. 2.
33 *Ibid*, p.3.
34 The College set up a Research Committee and started publishing a *Research Newsletter* in 1953. An 'Epidemic Observation Scheme' was started in 1954.
35 College Research Committee, 'The continuing observation and recording of morbidity', *Journal of the College of General Practitioners*, vol. 1, 1958, p. 107.
36 S.E. England Faculty, 'Report on epidemic winter vomiting', *College of General Practitioners' Research Newsletter*, no. 8, 1955, p. 96.
37 S.W. England Faculty, 'Report on obstetric survey', *College of General Practitioners' Research Newsletter*, no. 10, 1956, p. 24.
38 Yorkshire Faculty, 'Report on survey of unrecorded cases of cancer', *College of General Practitioners' Research Newsletter*, no. 13, 1956, p. 183.
39 B. Finlay et al., 'Stress and distress in general practice', *Practitioner*, vol. 172, 1954, p. 183.
40 J. Horder & E. Horder, 'Illness in general practice', *Practitioner*, vol. 173, 1954, p. 177.
41 J. Fry, 'Five years of general practice: a study in simple epidemiology', *British Medical Journal*, vol. 2, 1957, p. 1453.
42 E.M. Backett et al., 'Studies of general practice', *Proceedings of the Royal Society of Medicine*, vol. 46, 1953, p. 707.
43 D.L. Crombie, 'Prevalence of psychogenic illness in general practice', *College of General Practitioners' Research Newsletter*, no. 16, 1957, p. 218.
44 R.N. Theakston, 'A social survey in a country practice', *College of General Practitioners' Research Newsletter*, no. 16, 1957, p. 228.
45 R.P.C. Handfield-Jones, 'One year's work in a country practice', *Journal of the College of General Practitioners*, vol. 2, 1959, p. 323.
46 J.G. Bancroft & C.A.H. Watts, 'A survey of patients with chronic illness in general practice', *Journal of the College of General Practitioners*, vol. 2, 1959, p. 338.
47 D.L. Crombie, 'A casualty survey', *Journal of the College of General Practitioners*, vol. 2, 1959, p. 346.
48 C.A.H. Watts, 'The GP and research', *Journal of the College of General Practitioners*, vol. 1, suppl., 1958, p. 37.
49 *Ibid*, p. 39.
50 There is no necessary congruence between the levels of discourse, effects and practices, as Gordon has pointed out: C. Gordon (ed.), *Michel Foucault: power/knowledge*, Brighton, Harvester, 1980.
51 *General practice and the training of the general practitioner*, British Medical Association, 1950.
52 Report of the General Practice Steering Committee, 'A college of general practitioners', *British Medical Journal*, vol. 2, 1952, p. 1321.

53 C.R.G. Howard, 'The problem of defining the extent of morbidity in general pactice', *Journal of the College of General Practitioners*, vol. 2, 1959, p. 119.

54 R.J.F.H. Pinsent, 'Research in general practice', *Journal of the College of General Practitioners*, vol. 1, 1958, p. 23.

55 M. Marcus, 'The patient as a whole person. The problem of stress in general practice', *Journal of the College of General Practitioners*, vol. 1, suppl. no. 2, 1958, p. 26.

56 See for example, I. Pirrie, 'The GP at the crossroads', *British Medical Journal*, vol. 2, 1950, p. 169 L. Johnston, 'Preparing for general practice', *Lancet*, vol. 2, 1950, p. 824; W.M.E. Anderson, 'The GP at the crossroads', *British Medical Journal*, vol. 1, 1950, p. 1437.

In a previous paper I ascribed the emergence of complaints about trivia to a concern about the low status of the GP's work vis-a-vis that of hospital medicine without recognising that these complaints belonged to a general discourse on trivia, both 'negative' and 'positive', which emerged at this time: D. Armstrong, 'The emancipation of biographical medicine', *Social Science and Medicine*, vol. 13, 1979, p. 1.

57 M. Lask, 'The GP at the crossroads', *British Medical Journal*, vol. 1, 1950, p. 902.

58 L. Johnston, 'Preparing for general practice'.

59 Editorial, 'Diagnosis and nosology of minor maladies', *College of General Practitioners' Research Newsletter*, no. 6, 1955, p. 5.

60 See for example, J. Fry, 'A year of general practice'.

61 Suggested by the Statistics Sub-Committee of the Registrar-General's Advisory Committee on Medical Nomenclature and Statistics, *Measurement of morbidity*.

62 Pointed out as a problem, for example, by C.R.G. Howard, 'Defining the extent of morbidity', p. 122.

63 J. Horder & E. Horder, 'Illness in general practice', p. 184.

64 E.M. Backett et al., 'Studies of general practice'.

65 See, for example, D. Mechanic & E.H. Volkart, 'Illness behaviour and medical diagnoses', *Journal of Health and Human Behaviour*, vol. 1, 1960, p. 86; and D. Mechanic, 'The concept of illness behaviour', *Journal ofChronic Diseases*, vol. 15, 1962, p. 189.

66 See, for example, M.E.J. Wadsworth et al., *Health and sickness: The choice of treatment*, London, Tavistock, 1971.

67 See, for example, the early writings on the 'validity' of patients' symptoms, either in terms of their identification or in terms of external medical referrents, e.g., D. Mechanic & M. Newton, 'Some problems in the analysis of morbidity data', *Journal of Chronic Disease*, vol. 18, 1965, p. 569; and E.A. Suchman & B.S. Phillips, 'An analysis of the validity of health questionaires', *Social Forces*, vol. 36, 1958, p. 223.

The disappearance of these methodological issues takes place when, in the late 1970s, the whole field of illness behaviour is removed from the centre of medical sociologists' research interests. A workshop at the Annual Conference of the Medical Sociology Group in 1976, was on the question: 'Whatever happened to illness behaviour?'

68 All quotations taken from Discussion: 'What is general practice?', *Proceedings of the Royal Society of Medicine*, vol. 44, 1951, p. 113.

69 C.A.H. Watts, 'The GP and research'.

70 D. O'Neill, 'Stress problems in general practice', *Journal of the College of General Practitioners*, vol. 1, suppl. no. 2, 1958, p. 7.

71 M. Marcus, 'The patient as a whole person', *ibid*, p. 10.

72 See for example, J.H. Hunt, 'The scope and development of general practice in relation to other branches of medicine', *Lancet*, vol. 2, 1955, p. 681; or L.W. Batten, 'The essence of general practice', *Lancet*, vol. 2, 1956, p. 365.

73 J.H. Hunt, 'The scope and development of general practice'.

74 See, for example, P. Hopkins, 'Psychotherapy in general practice', *Lancet*, vol. 2, 1955, p. 455 C.A.H. Watts, *Neuroses in general practice*, London, Constable, 1956; H.S. Pasmore, 'Psychiatry in general practice', *Lancet*, vol. 1, 1958, p. 524 C.A.H. Watts, 'Management of chronic psychoneurosis in general practice', *Lancet*, vol. 2, 1958, p. 362.

75 M. Balint, 'The doctor, his patient and the illness', *Lancet*, vol. 1, p. 683, 1955, later published as book with same title: London, Pitman, 1956.

76 *Ibid.*

77 J. Horder, 'The role of the GP in psychological medicine', *Proceedings of the Royal Society of Medicine*, vol. 60, 1967, p. 264.

78 Consultative Council on Medical and Allied Services, *Interim report on the future provision of medical and allied services* (Dawson Report), London, HMSO, 1920; see also chapter 4 of this book.

79 'It shall be the duty of every local authority to provide, equip and maintain to the satisfaction of the Minister premises which shall be called health centres.' Section 21, *National Health Service Act*, London, HMSO, 1946.

80 H.W. Ashworth, 'The failure of health centres', *Journal of the College of General Practitioners*, vol. 2 1959, p. 357.

81 For an account of this period, see, J.G. Beales, *Sick health centres*, London, Pitman, 1978, pp. 13–14.

82 *Ibid.*

83 Ten health centres were in existence before the NHS. 23 were opened in the years 1948–65 60 were opened during 1966–8: M. Clarke, 'Health centres: an evaluation of past and present developments', *Update*, vol. 5, 1972, p. 1185.

A renewed interest in health centres can be identified from the late 1950s onwards, e.g., H.W. Ashworth, 'The failure of health centres'; Editorial, 'Health centres or medical centres?', *Lancet*, vol. 1, 1961, p. 149.

84 J.R. Edwards, '*A survey of health centres in the south-west*', Update publications, 1972. Reported in D. Hicks, *Primary health care*, London, HMSO, 1976.

85 For an overview see C. Watson & M. Clarke, 'Attachment schemes and development of the health care team', *Update*, vol. 5, 1972, p. 489.

86 Report of the Sub-Committee of the Standing Medical Advisory Committee, CHSC, *The field of work of the family doctor*, London, HMSO, 1963 (Gillie Report).

87 C. Watson & M. Clarke, 'Health centres'.

88 Gillie Report.

89 'The family doctor service: a Charter from the BMA', *Lancet*, vol. 1, 1965, p. 594.
90 M. Drury, 'Work-load and the general practitioner', *Lancet*, vol. 2, 1967, p. 823.
91 J. Fry, 'Administration and the general practitioner', *Lancet*, vol. 2, 1967, p. 1193.
92 *Ibid.*

Chapter 9

1 For history, see, for example, J.H. Howell, *A student's guide to geriatrics*, London, Staples Press, 1963, chapter 1.
2 J.H. Sheldon, *The social medicine of old age*, Oxford, Nuffield, 1948.
3 B. Seebohm Rowntree, *Old people: a report of the Survey Committee on the problem of ageing and the care of old people*, Oxford, Nuffield, 1947.
4 J.H. Sheldon, 'Some aspects of old age', *Lancet*, vol. 1, 1948, p. 621.
5 J.H. Sheldon, 'The social medicine of old age', p. 8.
6 *Ibid.*
7 W. Hobson & J. Pemberton, *The health of the elderly at home*, London, Butterworth, 1955.
8 A.P. Thompson et al., *The care of the ageing and chronic sick*, Edinburgh, Livingstone, 1951.
9 T. Ferguson, 'Aged sick nursed at home', *Lancet*, vol. 1, 1948, p. 417.
10 W. Hobson, 'General problems of ageing', in W. Hobson (ed.), *Modern trends in geriatrics*, London, Butterworth, 1956, p. 17.
11 J.H. Sheldon, quoted in *Report of the 3rd Congress of the International Association of Gerontology, London*, Edinburgh, Livingstone, 1954, p. 340.
12 J. Agate, *The practice of geriatrics*, London, Heinemann, 1963, p. 12.
13 T.H. Howell, *A student's guide to geriatrics*, p. 19.
14 T.H. Howell, *Old age: some practical points in geriatrics*, London, Lewis, 1975, p. 11.
15 *Ibid*, p. 165.
16 See, for example, J.C. Brocklehurst, *A textbook of geriatric medicine and gerontology*, London, Churchill Livingstone, 1973.
17 J.C. Brocklehurst, 'The elderly sick', *Lancet*, vol. 2, 1971, p. 657.
18 For a more detailed analysis see W.R. Arney & B.J. Bergen, 'The anomaly, the chronic patient and the play of medical power', *Sociology of Health and Illness*, forthcoming.
19 See, for example, N. Coni et al., *Lecture notes on geriatrics*, Oxford, Blackwell, 1977, p. 6.
20 F. Anderson, *Practical management of the elderly*, Oxford, Blackwell, 1967, p. 81.
21 *Ibid*, p. 403.
22 *Ibid*, p. 55.
23 G.R. Andrews et al., The 'practice of geriatric medicine in the community', in G. McLachlan (ed.), *Problems and progress in medical care, 5th series*, London, Nuffield, 1971.
24 M. Foucault, *The birth of the clinic: an archeology of medical perception*, London, Tavistock, 1963, pp. 16–20.

25 *Ibid*, p. 17.
26 J. Agate, *The practice of geriatrics*, p. 552.
27 See, for example, F. Anderson, *Practical management of the elderly*, chapter 24.
28 This tension between home and hospital is also apparent in the care of the dying: the recent 'hospice movement', for example, in a sense offers a medicalised space yet a natural death. See my earlier paper, D. Armstrong, 'Pathological life and death: medical spatialisation and geriatrics', *Social Science and Medicine*, vol. 15, 1981, p. 253. Much of the following section on the problem of the normal in geriatrics is drawn from it.
29 J. Agate, *The practice of geriatrics*, p. 40.
30 I. Felstein, *Later life: geriatrics today and tomorrow*, London, Penguin, 1969, p. 24.
31 F.I. Caird & T.G. Judge, *Assessment of the elderly*, London, Pitman, 1974, p. vii.
32 W. Hobson & J. Pemberton, *The health of the elderly at home*, pp. 23, 194.
33 A. Jordan, 'Normal values and the interpretation of biochemical data in the elderly', in W. Hobson, (ed.), *Modern trends in geriatrics.*
34 *Ibid.*
35 N. Coni et al., *Lecture notes in geriatrics*, p. 88.
36 S.C.D. Cayley, 'Care of the elderly', *Lancet*, vol. 1, 1976, p. 912.
37 B. Lush, 'The scope of research in geriatric medicine', *Age and Ageing*, vol. 3, 1974, p. 2.
38 M.K. Thompson, 'Can geriatrics survive?', *British Medical Journal*, vol. 1, 1976, p. 1590.
39 B. Lush, 'The scope of research in geriatric medicine'.
40 'One foot is the basic science or sciences that comprise gerontology and the other foot is clinical experience drawn from medicine in general.': R.I.S. Bayliss, 'Geriatrics and medical education', in J. Agate (ed), *Medicine in old age*, London, Pitman, 1966.
41 A.N. Exton-Smith, *Medical problems of old age*, Bristol, John Wright, 1955.
42 *Ibid.*
43 J. Agate, 'The practice of geriatrics', p. 11.
44 B. Isaacs, *An introduction to geriatrics*, London, Bailliere Tindall, 1965.
45 R.E. Tunbridge, 'Senescence, health and disease', in J. Agate (ed), *Medicine in old age.*
46 F. Anderson, *Practical management of the elderly*, p. 1.
47 *Ibid*, p. 20.
48 W.F. Anderson, 'Normal and abnormal ageing', in W.F. Anderson & B. Isaacs (eds), *Current achievements in geriatrics*, London, Cassell, 1964.
49 W.F. Anderson, *Practical management of the elderly*, p. 20.
50 N. Coni et al., *Lecture notes in geriatrics*, p. 88.
51 G. Adams, *Essentials of geriatric medicine*, London, Oxford University Press, 1977, p. 2.
52 J.H. Sheldon, 'Some aspects of old age'.
53 Lord Amulree, quoted in Editorial, 'Old and ailing', *Lancet*, vol. 1, 1947. p. 105.
54 B. Isaacs, 'Has geriatrics advanced?', in B. Isaacs (ed.), *Recent advances in geriatrics*, London, Churchill Livingstone, 1978. p. 2.

Chapter 10

1 *Report of the Inter-Departmental Committee on Medical Schools* (Ch., Goodenough), London, HMSO, 1944.
2 J.N. Morris, *Uses of epidemiology*, Edinburgh, Livingstone, 1957.
3 *Ibid*, p. 3.
4 *Ibid*, p. 40.
5 J.N. Morris, 'A medical examination of 1592 workers', *Lancet*, vol. 1, 1941, p. 51.
6 Medical Research Council, *Haemoglobin levels in Great Britain in 1943*, MRC Special Report no. 252, London, HMSO, 1945.
7 H.E. Magee & E.H.M. Milligan, 'Haemoglobin levels before and after labour', *British Medical Journal*, vol. 2, 1951, p. 1307.
8 W.T.C. Berry & H.E. Magee, 'Haemoglobin levels in adults and children', *British Medical Journal*, vol. 1, 1952, p. 410.
9 A.L. Cochrane et al., 'Pulmonary tuberculosis in the Rhondda Fach: an interim report of a survey of a mining community', *British Medical Journal*, vol. 2, 1952, p. 843.
10 I.T.T. Higgins et al., 'Respiratory symptoms and pulmonary disability in an industrial town: survey of a random sample of the population', *British Medical Journal*, vol. 2, 1956, p. 904.
11 College of General Pactitioners, 'Chronic bronchitis in Great Britain', *British Medical Journal*, vol. 2, 1961, p. 973.
12 V.A. Getting et al., 'Evaluation of a method of self-testing for diabetes', *Diabetes*, vol. 1, 1952, p. 194.
13 R.E. Tunbridge, 'Sociomedical aspects of diabetes mellitus', *Lancet*, vol. 2, 1953, p. 893.
14 I. Redhead, 'Incidence of glycosuria and diabetes mellitus in a general practice', *British Medical Journal*, vol. 1, 1960, p. 695.
15 J.B. Walker & D. Kerridge, *Diabetes in an English community*, Leicester University Press, 1961.
16 J. Harkness, 'Prevalence of glycosuria and diabetes mellitus: a comprehensive survey in an urban community', *British Medical Journal*, vol. 1, 1962, p. 1503.
17 Report of a working party appointed by the College of General Practitioners, 'A diabetes survey', *British Medical Journal*, vol. 1, 1962, p. 1497.
18 See, for example, 'Diabetes survey: Bedford 1962', *Proceedings of the Royal Society of Medicine*, vol. 57, 1964, p. 193.
19 R. Doll et al., 'Occupational factors in the aetiology of gastric and duodenal ulcers', *Special Report Series of the Medical Research Council, no. 276*, London, HMSO, 1951.
20 A.M. Stewart & J.P.W. Hughes, 'Mass radiography findings in the Northamptonshire boot and shoe industry, 1945–6', *British Medical Journal*, vol. 1, 1951, p. 899.
21 See, for example, W.E. Miall et al., 'An epidemiological study of rheumatoid arthritis associated with characteristic chest x-ray appearances in coal-workers', *British Medical Journal*, vol. 2, 1953, p. 1231.

22 M. Hamilton, G. Pickering et al., 'The aetiology of essential hypertension', *Clinical Science*, vol. 13, 1954, p. 11.
23 J.N. Morris, *Uses of epidemiology.*
24 *Ibid*, p. 70.
25 L.J. Witts (ed.), *Medical surveys and clinical trials*, London, Oxford University Press, 1959.
26 *Ibid*, p. 11.
27 H. Keen, 'Presymptomatic diagnosis of diabetes', *Proceedings of the Royal Society of Medicine*, vol. 59, 1966, p. 1169.
28 *Ibid.*
29 K. Faber, *Nosography in modern internal medicine*, London, Oxford University Press, 1923.
30 F.G. Crookshank (ed.), *Influenza: essays by several authors*, London, Heinemann, 1922.
31 L.S. King, 'What is disease?', *Philosophy of Science*, vol. 21, 1954, p. 194.
32 W. Riese, *The conception of disease: its history, its versions and its nature*, New York, Philosophical Library, 1953, p. 89.
33 J.A. Ryle, *Changing disciplines*, London, Oxford University Press, 1948.
34 *Ibid.*
35 H. Cohen, 'The evolution of the concept of disease', *Proceedings of the Royal Society of Medicine*, vol. 48, 1955, pp. 162, 167.
36 M. Hamilton et al., 'The aetiology of essential hypertension'.
37 G. Pickering, 'Logic and hypertension', *Lancet*, vol. 2, 1962, p. 149.
38 M. Hamilton et al., 'The aetiology of essential hypertension'.
39 *Ibid.*
40 J. McMichael, 'Logic and hypertension', *Lancet*, vol. 2, 1962, p. 99.
41 'Diabetes survey: Bedford 1962', *Proceedings of the Royal Society of Medicine*, vol. 57, 1964, p. 193.
42 See, for example, L. Breslow, 'Multiphasic screening in California', *Journal of Chronic Diseases*, vol. 2, 1955, p. 375; and M.L. Levin, 'Screening for asymptomatic disease', *Journal of Chronic Diseases*, vol. 2, 1955, p. 367.
43 See, for example, R.J. Donaldson & J.M. Howell, 'A multiple screening clinic', *British Medical Journal*, vol. 2, 1965, p. 1034.
44 *Screening in medical care: reviewing the evidence*, London, Nuffield, 1968.
45 W.J.H. Butterfield, *Priorities in medicine*, London, Nuffield, 1968.
46 J.N. Morris, *Uses of epidemiology* (2nd edn).
47 J.N. Morris, *Uses of epidemiology* (1st edn), p. 66.
48 J.A. Ryle, 'Aetiology: a plea for wider concepts and new study', *Lancet*, vol. 2, 1942, p. 29.
49 *Ibid.*
50 R. Muir, *Textbook of pathology*, London, Arnold, 1933 (3rd edn).
51 *Ibid.*
52 *Ibid* (6th edn), 1951.
53 *Ibid* (5th edn), 1941.
54 *Ibid.*
55 *Ibid.*

56 J.A. Ryle, 'Aetiology: a plea for wider concepts'.
57 E. Durkheim, *Elementary forms of the religious life*, London, Allen and Unwin, 1933.
58 J.A. Ryle, 'Aetiology: a plea for wider concepts', p. 30.
59 D. MacKay, *Hospital morbidity statistics: studies on medical and population subjects*, London, HMSO, 1951.

Chapter 11

1 T. McKeown, *Medicine in modern society*, London, Allen and Unwin, 1965, p. 177.
2 Report of the Committee on Child Health Services, *Fit for the future* (Court Report), London, HMSO, 1976.
3 See, for example, Editorial, 'General practitioners and psychiatrists – a new relationship?', *Journal of the Royal College of General Practitioners*, vol. 28, 1978, p. 643.
4 See, for example, L. Kanner, 'Trends in child psychiatry', *Journal of Mental Science*, vol. 105, 1959, p. 581.
5 See, for example, papers by T.H.D. Arie & M. Roth, in G. McLachlan (ed.), *Approaches to action: a symposium on service for the mentally ill and handicapped*, London, Nuffield, 1972.
6 *Report of the Inter-Departmental Committee on Medical Schools* (Goodenough Report), London, HMSO, 1944.
7 *Ibid*, p. 140.
8 *Ibid*, p. 157.
9 *Report of the Royal Commission on Medical Education* (Todd Report), London, HMSO, 1968.
10 *Ibid*, p. 11.
11 A.D. Frazer, 'The problem of the defaulter', *British Journal of Venereal Diseases*, vol. 8, 1932, p. 56.
12 *Ibid*. p. 58.
13 M. Foucault, *Discipline and punish: the birth of the prison*, London, Allen Lane, 1978, see part III.
14 Hanschell, H.M. 'The defaulting seaman', *British Journal of Venereal Diseases*, vol. 11, 1935, p. 28.
15 H. Nichol, 'The defaulting prostitute', *ibid*, p. 31.
16 H. Nichol, 'The defaulting travelling man', *ibid*, p. 98.
17 D. Nabarro, 'The defaulting child', *ibid*, p. 91.
18 W.V. McFarlane & H.M. Johns, 'The problem of default in a venereal diseases clinic: a medico–social analysis of 381 women patients', *British Journal of Venereal Diseases*, vol. 23, 1947, p. 171.
19 P. Ley, 'Towards better doctor–patient communications', in A.E. Bennett (ed.), *Communication between doctors and patients*. London, Nuffield, 1976.
20 *Ibid*, p. 82.
21 See chapter 3 of this book.
22 L. Cole, 'Prognosis and the patient', *Lancet*, vol. 1, 1946, p. 1.
23 T.G. Armstrong, 'The use of reassurance', *Lancet*, vol. 2, 1946, p. 480.
24 J. Parkinson, 'The patient and the physician', *Lancet*, vol. 2, 1951, p. 457.

25 A. Meares, 'Communication and the patient', *Lancet*, vol. 1, 1960, p. 663.
26 Joint Sub-Committee of the Standing Medical and Standing Nursing Advisory Committees for the Central Health Services Council, *Communication between doctors, nurses and patients: an aspect of human relations in the hospital service*, London, HMSO, 1963.
27 *Ibid*, p. 7.
28 Editorial, 'Human relations in hospital', *Lancet*, vol. 2, 1963, p. 77.
29 A. Cartwright, *Human relations and hospital care*, London, Routledge and Kegan Paul, 1964.
30 C.M. Fletcher, *Communication in medicine*, London, Nuffield, 1973.
31 *Ibid*, p. 17.
32 H.B. Brackenbury, *Patient and doctor*, London, Hodder and Stoughton, 1935, p. 72.
33 F. Honigsbaum, *The division in British medicine*, London, Kogan Page, 1979, p. 146.
34 H.B. Brackenbury, *Patient and doctor*, p. 74.
35 *Ibid*, p. 77.
36 *Ibid*, p. 109.
37 *Ibid*, p. 100.
38 M.P. Raven, 'Medicine as an art', *Lancet*, vol. 2, 1932, p. 602.
39 C.M. Campbell, 'The GP's approach to his nervous and mental patients', *British Medical Journal*, vol. 2, 1932, p. 1186.
40 H. Crichton-Miller, 'Primitive man and the modern patient', *British Medical Journal*, vol. 2, 1932, p. 430.
41 E. Jones, 'The unconscious mind and medical practice', *British Medical Journal*, vol. 1, 1938, p. 1354.
42 H. Lett, 'The entrance into medicine', *British Medical Journal*, vol. 1, 1939, p. 1190.
43 M. Cassidy, 'Doctor and patient', *Lancet*, vol. 1, 1938, p. 175.
44 E.D. Wittkower, 'Psychological aspects of venereal disease', *British Journal of Venereal Diseases*, vol. 24, 1948, p. 59.
45 *Ibid*, p. 62.
46 R. Sutherland, 'Some individual and social factors in venereal disease', *British Journal of Venereal Diseases*, vol. 25, 1950, p. 1.
47 Planning Committee of the Royal College of Physicians, *Report on medical education*, London, RCP 1944.
48 *Ibid*, p. 22.
49 *Ibid*, p. 25.
50 *Ibid*, p. 31.
51 J. Spence, 'The need for understanding the individual as part of the training and function of doctors and nurses', 1949 lecture. Reprinted in J. Spence, *The purpose and practice of medicine*, London, Oxford University Press, 1960.
52 H. Cairns, 'The student's objective', *Lancet*, vol. 2, 1949, p. 665.
53 M. Balint, 'The doctor, his patient and the illness', *Lancet*, vol. 1, 1955, p. 683.
54 M. Balint, *The doctor, his patient and the illness*, London, Pitman, 1956.

55 K.A.J. Järvinen, 'Can ward rounds be a danger to patients with myocardial infarcation?', *British Medical Journal*, vol. 1, 1955, p. 318.
56 R.M. Ellison, 'Strained relations', *Lancet*, vol. 2, 1955, p. 1330.
57 A.E. Clark-Kennedy, 'Medicine in relation to society', *British Medical Journal*, vol. 1, 1955, p. 619.
58 H.L. Rogerson, 'Venereophobia in the male', *British Journal of Venereal Diseases*, vol. 26, 1951, p. 158.
59 Venereologists Group Committee, 'Social work in the venereal disease service', *British Journal of Venereal Diseases*, vol. 28, 1952, p. 146.
60 G.O. Horne, 'The contemporary defaulter in the venereal disease clinic – further observations', *British Journal of Venereal Diseases*, vol. 29, 1953, p. 210.
61 J. O'Hare, 'The road to promiscuity', *British Journal of Venereal Diseases*, vol. 36, 1960, p. 122.
62 *Ibid*, p. 124.
63 K. Browne & P. Freeling, 'The doctor–patient relationship', *Practitioner*, vol. 196, pp. 168, 316, 454, 730, 868 vol. 197, pp. 112, 252, 1966.
64 K. Browne & P. Freeling. *The doctor–patient relationship*, London, Churchill Livingstone, 1967.
65 *Ibid*, p. 1.
66 *The future general practitioner*, London, Royal College of General Practitioners, 1972.
67 P. Hopkins, *Patient-centred medicine*, London, Regional Doctor Publication, 1972.
68 R. Hutchison & H. Rainy, *Clinical methods*, London, Cassel, 1897 (1st edn).
69 R. Hutchison & D. Hunter, *Clinical methods*, London, Cassel, 1949 (12th edn).
70 R. Bomford et al., *Hutchison's clinical methods*, London, Bailliere Tindall, 1975 (16th edn).
71 *Ibid*.
72 M. Foucault, *Discipline and punish*, p. 192.
73 See, for example, W.R. Arney, *Power and the profession of obstetrics*, Chicago University Press, forthcoming.
74 C. Gordon (ed), *Michel Foucault: power/knowledge*, Brighton, Harvester, 1980, p. 96.
75 M. Foucault, *Discipline and punish*, p. 138.

Chapter 12

1 M. Foucault, *Discipline and punish: the birth of the prison*, London, Allen Lane, 1977, p. 193.
2 T. Parsons, *The social system*, New York, Free Press, 1951, chapter 10.
3 H. Brackenbury, *Doctor and patient*, London, Hodder, 1935.
4 E. Freidson, 'Dilemmas in the doctor–patient relationship', first published in 1961. Reprinted in A.M. Rose (ed.), *Human behaviour and social processes*, London, Routledge and Kegan Paul 1962.
5 T. Szasz & M. Hollander, 'The basic models of the doctor–patient relationship', *Archives of Internal Medicine*, vol. 97, 1956, p. 585.
6 M. Balint, *The doctor, his patient and the illness*, London, Pitman, 1956.

7 E. Freidson, *Profession of Medicine*, New York, Dodds Mead, 1970.
8 K. Browne & P. Freeling, *The doctor–patient relationship*, London, Churchill Livingstone, 1967.
9 G. Stimson & B. Webb, *Going to see the doctor*, London, Routledge and Kegan Paul, 1975.
10 E. Rubington & M.S. Weinberg, *Deviance: the inter-actionist perspective*, London, Collier–Macmillan, 1968.
11 G. Stimson & B. Webb, *Going to see the doctor*, p. 8.
12 See, for example, M. Wadsworth & D. Robinson, *Studies in every-day medical life*, London, Martin Robertson, 1976.
13 N. Jewson, 'Disappearance of the sick-man from medical cosmologies, 1770–1870', *Sociology*, vol. 10, 1976, p. 225.
14 K. Figlio, 'The historiography of scientific medicine', *Comparative Studies in Society and History*, vol. 19, 1977, p. 262.
15 C. Gordon (ed.), *Michel Foucault: power/knowledge*, Brighton, Harvester, 1980, p. 239.
16 *Ibid.* p. 58.
17 M. Foucault, *Discipline and punish*, p. 192.

Index